ALTERNATIVES IN REHABILITATING
THE HANDICAPPED

ALTERNATIVES IN REHABILITATING THE HANDICAPPED

A Policy Analysis

Edited by
Jeffrey Rubin, Ph. D.

Rutgers University
New Brunswick,
New Jersey

with
Valerie LaPorte, M.A., M. Phil.
RELEASED

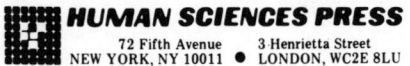
HUMAN SCIENCES PRESS
72 Fifth Avenue   3 Henrietta Street
NEW YORK, NY 10011 ● LONDON, WC2E 8LU

Copyright © 1982 by Human Sciences Press
72 Fifth Avenue, New York, New York 10011

All rights reserved. No part of this work may be reproduced or utilized in any form or by any means, electronic of manual, including photocopying, microfilm and recording, or by any information storage and retrieval system without permission in writing from the publisher.

Printed in the United States of America
123456789   987654321

Editorial/Production Services
by **Harkavy Publishing Service**

Library of Congress Cataloging in Publication Data

Main entry under title:

Alternatives in rehabilitating the handicapped.

Includes bibliographical references and index.
1. Vocational rehabilitation—Addresses, essays, lectures.   I. Rubin, Jeffrey, 1949– . II. LaPorte, Valerie.   [DNLM: 1. Rehabilitation, Vocational—Trends—United States.   HD 7256.U5 A711]
HD7255.A47   362'.0425   81-4144
ISBN 0-89885-010-X   AACR2

CONTENTS

Contributors   vii

List of Tables   ix

Preface   xi

Acknowledgments   xiii

Introduction   xv
    Monroe Berkowitz and Jeffrey Rubin

1. An Economic Evaluation of the Beneficiary Rehabilitation Program   **1**
    Monroe Berkowitz, Martin Horning, Stephen McConnell, Jeffrey Rubin and John D. Worrall

2. Rehabilitation, Employment and the Disabled   **89**
    Sar Levitan and Robert Taggart

3. Vocational Rehabilitation Perspectives for Policy Analysis and Change   **151**
    Marvin Sussman

4. Predicting Future Disability and Rehabilitation
   Policies in the United States form the Northwestern
   European Experience   189
   John H. Noble, Jr.

5. Private and Public Rehabilitation   215
   George T. Welsh

6. Rehabilitation of the Severely Handicapped,
   PL 93-112: A Retrospective Appraisal by a State
   Vocational Rehabilitation Director   229
   Donald E. Galvin

CONTRIBUTORS

Monroe Berkowitz is professor of economics at Rutgers College. He is coauthor of *Public Policy Toward Disability*, Praeger, 1976 and many other studies on the economics of disability policy.

Donald E. Galvin, at the time of the seminar on which the volume is based, was the Associate Superintendent of Education and Director of the Michigan Bureau of Rehabilitation. At present, he is a professor of Rehabilitation Counseling and Community Health Sciences and director of the University Center for International Rehabilitation at Michigan State University. He was selected as a fellow for the 1980 Mary Switzer Memorial Lecture and was recently appointed to the National Council on the Handicapped.

Martin Horning is an assistant professor of economics at Mount Union College, Mount Union, Ohio. He has received the Military Order of the Purple Heart's Award for Outstanding Research in Services to the Handicapped for his dissertation, "Nondisabled-Disabled Wage Differentials: An Empirical Test for Discrimination."

Valerie LaPorte is a doctoral candidate in the Department of English at Columbia University. She is currently teaching at the Newark campus of Rutgers University. She is coeditor of *Reform and Regulation in Long-Term Care*, Praeger, 1979.

Sar A. Levitan is Research Professor of Economics and Director of the Center for Social Policy Studies at the George Washington University. He served as chairman of the National Commission on Employment and Unemployment Statistics. Professor Levitan has authored or coauthored numerous articles and books, including *Human Resources and Labor Markets* and *Programs in Aid for the Poor*.

Stephen McConnell was formerly a research associate in the Disability and Health Economics Research Section at Rutgers. He is coauthor of *Uniform Data Systems and Related Subjects in Workers' Compensation*, Volume 2 of the Research Report of the Interdepartmental Workers' Compensation Task Force.

Jim Noble is a program analyst with the Office of the Assistant Secretary for Planning and Budget in the Department of Education. His articles have appeared in *Evaluation Quarterly* and *The Journal of Health Politics, Policy, and the Law*.

Jeffrey Rubin is an assistant professor of economics at Rutgers College. He is the author of *Economics, Mental Health, and the Law*, Lexington Books, D.C. Heath, 1978.

Marvin B. Sussman is Unidel Professor of Human Behavior in the College of Human Resources, University of Delaware. He has published and written numerous articles and books, as well as serving as editor for the journal, *Marriage and Family Review* and associate editor for the *Journal of Marriage and Family Therapy* and *The Journal of Marriage and Family*. He is the 1980 recipient of the Ernest W. Burgess Award of the National Council on Family Relations.

Robert Taggart III is currently the director of the Youth Knowledge Development Project. He is formerly the Administrator of the Office of Youth Programs in the Employment and Training Administration of the Department of Labor.

George Welch is President of International Rehabilitation Associates Inc., a private rehabilitation firm. He has lectured throughout the world on insurance rehabilitation. Mr. Welch is a member of the board of directors and executive committee of Rehabilitation International-U.S.A. and was chairman of the U.S. delegation to the World Assembly on Rehabilitation at Ofir, Portugal.

John Worrall is Vice President and Director of Research at the National Council on Compensation Insurance. He is coauthor of *An Evaluation of Policy-Related Rehabilitation Research*, Praeger, 1975.

LIST OF TABLES

Chapter I

1-1	Number of Clients Served by State Vocational Rehabilitation Agencies by Type of Program	12
1-2	Number of Rehabilitations Reported by State Vocational Rehabilitation Agencies by Type of Program	12
1-3	Savings Through Terminations	21
1-4	Termination Savings with GAO Assumptions	22
1-5	Present Value of Savings and Costs	24
1-6	Hypothetical Illustration of Costs and Savings for One Client	28
1-7	Reallocation of Allotments According to Rehabilitations	36
1-8	Reallocation of Allotments According to Termination of 1973 BRP Rehabilitations	40
1-9	Reallocation of Allotments According to Savings to DI Trust Fund	46
1-10	Rudiments of An Ideal Financing Plan	53
1-11	Wages at Closure and Rate of Termination	62
1-12	Wage/Benefit Ratio and the Rate of Termination	64
1-13	Probability of Termination Regression Results White Male Cohort of 1973 BRP Rehabilitants	66

x ALTERNATIVES IN REHABILITATING THE HANDICAPPED

1-14	Probability of Termination Regression Results White Male Cohort of 1973 BRP Rehabilitants	68
1-15	Probability of Termination Regression Results White Male Cohort of 1973 BRP Rehabilitants With Wages at Closure Equal to or Greater Than the 1974 SGA Limit	70
1-16	Replacement Rates and Rates of Termination by Age Categories	79

Chapter 2

2-1	Vocational Rehabilitation Activity 1965 and 1975	91
2-2	Disabled Reporting Having Received Rehabilitation Services, 1966 and 1972	92
2-3	Source of Rehabilitation Services Received by Disabled, 1972	94

Chapter 4

4-1	Social Security System Compared, 1975	192
4-2	Variables Influencing the Outcomes of Rehabilitation	199
4-3	Ratio of Actual to Expected Claims by the Ratio of Gross Benefits to Salary: Group Long Term Disability Insurance with Six Month Deferment Period, North America, 1966–1972	200
4-4	Changes in Male and Female Populations, Ages 50–64, Their Labor Force Participation (LFP), and Resulting Increase or Decline as Ratio of Expected Value of Populations at End of Time Period, Selected Countries and Years	208

PREFACE

The collection of papers that constitutes this book is testimony to the diversity and complexity that characterize vocational rehabilitation. The papers were chosen to bring to the reader an understanding of these traits of vocational rehabilitation as well as to document the changes rehabilitation is undergoing as the program enters the 1980s. As if the analysis is not difficult enough, the issues will be further complicated as new clients enter the system and new objectives are formulated.

The authors, coming as they do from such a wide variety of disciplines with a similarly broad range of experiences, are well aware of the problems. Nonetheless, they share a common interest in the quality of rehabilitation programs. Their respect for past accomplishments and their individual views of the rehabilitation system do not guarantee that a consensus will exist on program goals, methods, or prospects. Yet the authors are in agreement, both among themselves and with legislators, administrators, counselors, and clients, that the search for ways to improve performance, to increase the availability of services, and to more equitably allocate limited resources must go on with renewed vigor.

The idea that spawned this and companion volumes on disability policy and long-term care was formulated in the Office of Social Services and Human Development (SSHD) in the Department of Health, Education, and Welfare. John Noble and John DeWilde commissioned a series of papers by experts in disability policy covering a broad range of issues. In addition, SSHD was continuing its sponsorship of other disability research at Rutgers. After the papers and research were completed, it became clear that some dissemination plan was necessary. Two approaches were taken: First, the Disability and Health Economics Research (DHER) Section at Rutgers and HEW co-sponsored a series of disability overview seminars, including one on rehabilitation. Second, it was decided to combine some of the overview papers in rehabilitation with the rehabilitation seminar presentations and some of the sponsored research. The result is the collection of papers in this volume.

Along the way a great many debts were incurred. Of course, our greatest debt is to the authors who persevered with us in the long gestation from commissioning the papers to seeing the book in print.

Valerie LaPorte of DHER was responsible for the copyediting of most of the papers. The variety of origins made her task a difficult one and yet the consistency and readability of the book are testimony to the quality of her effort.

Monroe Berkowitz, director of DHER, organized the seminars and oversaw the editing and production of the volume. Lynne Lavigne was indispensable in the management of the entire effort from drafts to dissemination of the final product.

ACKNOWLEDGMENTS

The preparation of this book was supported in part by a grant (HEW Grant 009A-7701, 02 and 03) from the Office of the Assistant Secretary for Planning and Evaluation, Office of Social Services and Human Development, Department of Health, Education and Welfare to the Disability and Health Economics Research Section of the Bureau of Economic Research, Rutgers University. Any findings, opinions, conclusions or recommendations expressed are those of the authors and do not necessarily reflect the views of HEW.

INTRODUCTION

Monroe Berkowitz and Jeffrey Rubin

The logic behind a vocational rehabilitation program is indisputable. It is far better to restore a man to a useful job than to see him languish unused and unwanted. It is far better to spend money to provide the medical restoration, training, counseling, guidance, and placement services to put him to work than to have him subsist on the public purse. It is on this basis that Congress has been willing to appropriate increasing amounts of money to finance a joint federal-state program of rehabilitation. Today that appropriation amounts to nearly one billion dollars each year. In addition, there are two specially financed rehabilitation programs: one for Social Security Disability Insurance (DI) recipients and one for Supplemental Security Income (SSI) recipients.

The rehabilitation program has always been dynamic.[1] In its beginnings, after World War I, the primary targets were the industrially injured who were receiving workers' compensation payments. In the next 30 years, other clients came into the program, but the crippled and orthopedically handicapped remained the primary recipients of vocational rehabilitation services. In the 1960s emphasis changed to include those who suffered from mental retardation and mental illness. During the "War on Poverty," the target shifted toward clients who were culturally disadvantaged. More recently, priority has been given to the severely disabled.

Because of its control of the purse and its responsibility to respond to public opinion, Congress has been and continues to be the agent on which the burden of policymaking in rehabilitation falls. Subject to pressures from many sides, Congress has enacted two far-reaching rehabilitation laws in the past six years. These legislative enactments, the Rehabilitation Act of 1973 and the Comprehensive Rehabilitation Services Amendments of 1978, are directed at changing three components of rehabilitation: client selection, rehabilitation method, and outcome objective.

In this volume, each of the authors is concerned with one or more of these components. Several threads link the papers: the importance of client incentives and circumstances, the interrelationship between the public and private sectors, the variables influencing counselor and agency performance, and the determination of program objectives.

Client incentives or what has been termed the disincentive issue is of primary concern. The expectation of severe work disincentives has long stymied efforts to reform the welfare system.[2] Recently, the question of incentives has begun to be encompassed in policy decisions in a broad range of social welfare programs.

Several explanations can be offered for this growing concern. Funding for social programs has become more vulnerable because of macro-fiscal problems. Efforts to balance the budget and reduce tax burdens have caused policymakers to investigate the benefits and costs of social programs more closely. As a result, some people have concluded that certain programs discourage employment and encourage certain possibly undesirable behaviors. One obvious example is the apparent excessive utilization of long-term care facilities by publicly insured individuals.[3]

At the program level, the failure of individual programs to perform up to expectation at a reasonable cost has also led to closer inspection. For example, even with growing welfare payments, the percentage of families remaining poor is substantial. Also, the current mix of public and private health protection has become very costly while gaps in coverage remain.[4] Evaluations have cast doubt on the performance of manpower and employment programs. As a result, there is a more skeptical and questioning attitude prevalent today with respect to such social programs.

One result of the shift in attitude toward social programs is that rehabilitation has become a target of critical analysis.[5] This volume represents a growing concern about how well rehabilitation works and more important, how it can be improved. It is encouraging to find areas of agreement on policy matters in the individual chapters. We will highlight policy options advanced by the individual authors. These can best be understood in light of recent legislation and possible future changes in the rehabilitation environment. In the following section we will briefly review recent rehabilitation legislation and analyze issues that rehabilitation personnel may have to deal with in the future. The introduction concludes with a more complete summary of the individual chapters.

POLICY OPTIONS IN THE PAPERS

It is not surprising to find questions being raised about incentives and disincentives in rehabilitation; in fact these are not new concerns.[6] But in this volume much new data and analysis are bought to bear on the issue. The role of disability benefit levels in reducing the incentive to rehabilitate is discussed by several of the authors. For a portion of the disabled, there is a disability-work status choice; high benefits can cause a greater amount of people to choose the former.[7]

Policy for dealing with disincentives can range from changing program format or altering benefit levels to improving rehabilitation performance, given whatever disincentives may exist. One suggestion, proposed by Berkowitz, Horning, McConnell, Rubin, and Worrall (see Chap. 1) is to improve selection of clients by making better use of knowledge about factors correlated with success. Sussman (see Chap. 3) shifts the focus to rehabilitation methods as a means to overcome disincentives. He suggests a closer linkage between an individual's family and his rehabilitation efforts. In his review, Noble (see Chap. 4) comments on another proposed change in method: immediate delivery of rehabilitation services before any disincentive effect takes hold.

Reforms designed to overcome disincentives are only one theme. Several commentators question the predominant role of public sector rehabilitation programs. Of late there has been a general trend toward reduced involvement of government in the lives of its citizens. Free market advocates believe there should be an increased role for private rehabilitation agencies.

The private versus public debate also affects rehabilitation with respect to employment. Private sector demands for labor in relation to the supply of labor can directly influence the willingness of employers to hire a disabled person. Recent legislation has also mandated affirmative action and nondiscrimination with regard to the handicapped population as well. At the same time, there appears to be a greater willingness to use the public sector to open up new job placements.[8]

Levitan and Taggart (see Chap. 2) see a close link between private market demand and rehabilitation success. On these grounds they see the program needing to concentrate its greatest efforts on vocational skills that will translate into success when the disabled seek employment in the private sector.

Welch (see Chap. 5) examines the public-private debate in terms of who will deliver services more efficiently. Citing a record of greater efficiency, he opts for an increased reliance on private rehabilitation efforts. Giving the market a chance to function is seen as leading to improved end results.

Where rehabilitation has not kept up with expectations public employment and quotas have been tried. Noble reviews these efforts elsewhere but is pessimistic about their chances for success in the United States.

Productivity in the public sector is another growing concern impinging on rehabilitation. Criticism directed at bureaucracy and its inefficiencies has led to calls for tighter control and greater accountability. But to talk of productivity and accountability requires a definition of both product and recipient. In the field of rehabilitation, the definitions of both have been changing.

Output in rehabilitation traditionally has been defined as employment in the competitive market. One exception is the Beneficiary Rehabilitation Program where termination of DI benefits is the ultimate goal. Termination requires not only employment but employment at a wage greater than that established as the substantial gainful activity level.

But the goal of a job in the competitive labor market as the traditional objective of a vocational rehabilitation program has been called into question. An improvement in independent living skills is becoming an acceptable outcome even though the concept is difficult to measure. Requirements for an individualized written rehabilitation plan (IWRP) are putting more pressure on counselors who are being told to serve the severely disabled and not those necessarily the most likely to complete the program successfully. As Noble notes, these incremental changes in client selection, methods, and outcomes are due to the political nature of rehabilitation financing and not to any well-conceived grand plan to improve rehabilitation efficiency.

The damage to effectiveness and to the overall performance of an agency is one of the themes of Galvin's chapter (see Chap. 6). He argues that agencies and counselors are being legislatively mandated to do things they are not equipped to do.

Our discussion of the problems and controversies in rehabilitation should not obscure their successes. In several of the chapters, empirical verification of the success of rehabilitation efforts is presented. But the programs will not be able to continue without change. Some of the change has improved performance as will some future changes currently under consideration.

The selection of clients, the methods of rehabilitation, and the objectives of the program undergo constant review and evaluation. In part, the changes that occur are a result of legislative action, and are forced on rehabilitation by outside events and circumstances. In the next section, we consider these origins of change in more detail.

SOME RECENT HISTORY AND PROSPECTS FOR THE FUTURE

This volume raises many issues about the current operation of rehabilitation programs. Some of the issues are inherently a part of any rehabilitation program while others are directly linked to the public rehabilitation program's legislative mandate. The concerns of rehabilitation in the next ten years will be jointly determined by both its inherent and legislative aspects.

On the legislative side are the controversial implications of the Rehabilitation Act of 1973. The priority accorded the severely disabled has brought into question the equity of the rehabilitation queue, the measurement of success, and the ability of agencies and counselors to adjust to the dictates of Congress. The requirement for an IWRP has led to greater involvement of the disabled themselves in planning their future, while at the same time, it has detracted from counselor autonomy and has required a considerable amount of resources. Along with these programmatic changes, the 1973 act mandated affirmative action for the handicapped and forbade discrimination against them by employers.

These changes keep the rehabilitation program up to date and responsive to client needs. At the same time, drastic changes such as these are not implemented overnight, nor are they free to everyone. We do not mean to imply that Congress has not recognized the consequences of the choices it has made; it is the responsibility of Congress to make these choices. But if their information is incomplete or their assumptions invalid, then research should be able to show the extent to which the costs or benefits of a particular component of legislation was inaccurately estimated. In rehabilitation, the legislative process has proved to be one that combines past program performance with changing circumstances in the development of new legislative initiatives.

Out of that process has emerged the most recent attempt to redesign public rehabilitation: The Comprehensive Rehabilitation Services Amendments of 1978. Just as the 1973 act ranged broadly in its attempt to restructure parts of the rehabilitation program, the drafters of the 1978 amendments sought to make major reforms in a variety of areas. One key element of the new amendments is a budget for basic state grants that is to be adjusted only in accordance with inflation, thus eliminating any real growth in the program through 1982. A limit on new spending reflects the general fiscal constraints faced by government and perhaps some doubts about the effectiveness of vocational rehabilitation.

A second important series of developments is the establishment of a National Institute of Handicapped Research (NIHR), to supplant the previous research apparatus, the creation of an interagency committee to improve the coordination of rehabilitation-related activities sponsored by various federal agencies and the establishment of a National Council on the Handicapped to set the policies of the NIHR and to oversee related rehabilitation programs.[9] The triumvirate of an institute, committee, and council may be indicative of Congressional dissatisfaction with the rehabilitation support activities. Whether they can more effectively relate research with service to the betterment of the program is not yet known.

The 1978 amendments added Section 505 to the Rehabilitation Act of 1973. One of its purposes was to encourage the application of the affirmative action and nondiscrimination sections (503 and 504 respectively) by allowing the courts to award attorney's fees to the prevailing party (other than the United States).

What will more than likely raise the greatest controversy are two new titles added to the Rehabilitation Act of 1973 by the

1978 amendments. Title VI, Part A, established in the Department of Labor a community service employment pilot program for handicapped people who are unlikely to find employment. Title VI, Part B, created a program to open up opportunities for handicapped individuals in industry by allowing the rehabilitation agencies to bear up to 80 percent of the costs involved in developing special on-the-job training programs.

The second new title, Title VII, authorizes grants to help states develop services for those severely disabled persons who currently lack the potential for employment. Instead of a vocational goal, services financed under Title VII would be directed toward helping the eligible population increase their ability to live and function independently.[10] The title signals a substantial departure from the traditional role of vocational rehabilitation and has generated a great deal of controversy. Along with questions as to whether independent living services should be part of the objectives of the rehabilitation process, there are doubts as to whether sufficient funds for the purposes spelled out in Title VII will be appropriated.

As the scope of these amendments suggest, the gaps and failings present in vocational rehabilitation have led to an enormously complex mix of actions and proposals. Whether the 1978 amendments will be implemented as their designers envisioned is yet to be answered, and we cannot know how well the changes will work even if put into practice. Changing circumstances and knowledge could well force a reevaluation of the new programs.

In both the distant and recent past, Congress and the rehabilitation community have not hesitated to offer reforms and as the 1978 amendments show, changes in rehabilitation can be quite dramatic. As the environment in which rehabilitation functions changes in the future, we should expect comparable changes in the direction of the programs. Four important areas where change may well influence the shape of future rehabilitation programs are the technology of rehabilitation, the financing of rehabilitation, the labor market demand for disabled workers, and the characteristics and behavior of the disabled themselves. Below we consider how each factor may change and how rehabilitation may be affected.

Technology of Rehabilitation

The technology of rehabilitation encompasses a broad range of possibilities embracing the restructuring of the method for delivering services as well as the kinds of services delivered. Examples include the development and application of mechanical technology, innovative uses of medical technology, and the redesign of our architectural environment.[11]

Both the impaired person and the environment in which he functions may be altered through the application of mechanical and other engineering devices. Sight, sound, and mobility are just a few of the capacities that can be improved through the use of technology. Counselors may be called upon to devote more time to the acquisition of knowledge about how new technologies can be directly applied by them for their clients' benefit.

With increasing judicial and legislative pressure on firms to employ the disabled, we can expect new and innovative uses of technology to modify the job and the job site. The ability of rehabilitation counselors to effectively utilize these private sector initiatives could greatly affect the success of their agencies.

Technology can also be of help in housing and transportation design. Eliminating man-made barriers is fundamental to rehabilitation success. Moreover, if rehabilitation programs take on a greater role in terms of improving daily living skills, there are likely to be any number of technologies that can be applied to the benefit of the disabled.

New developments in medical technology can lessen the impact of an impairment on an individual's functional ability and perhaps in the future overcome many of the most limiting aspects of impairments. At the same time, rehabilitation performance can be negatively affected by medical breakthroughs that prolong life but leave more individuals with a reduced capacity for independent functioning.

Finally there is what we might call the technology of using

technology. The utilization by rehabilitation counselors of existing and newly developed technology can be increased by improving the methods by which knowledge about these matters is transferred from researchers to users.

Financing

Financial rearrangements may be among the more effective alternatives to be used in the near future. Monetary incentives to states, counselors, disabled people, and businesses should all be tried. Linking rewards to successful rehabilitation is one way states and counselors can be encouraged to do the best possible job. At the same time, disabled persons are influenced by what are, in effect, substantial tax rates on earnings as they find employment. Attention must be paid to overcoming these disincentives and to encourage firms, perhaps through expanded use of tax credits for job modification, to increase employment of the handicapped. Alternatively, penalties charged against firms can be used to encourage private efforts to prevent an impaired worker from leaving his job and seeking disability status.

Labor Markets

A third factor that will influence rehabilitation performance is the functioning of labor markets. The ability of disabled persons to find employment depends both on their capabilities and the demands of employers for those skills. These employer demands in turn are a function of the demand for the product the firm is producing. Hence a strong economy makes it easier for counselors to place clients largely because firms are more interested in finding employees.

Given the prevailing economic uncertainties, ways to recession-proof rehabilitation efforts must be considered. Every attempt should be made to identify jobs for the disabled that are less subject to the fluctuations of the national economy. Although no one, particularly those recently hired, is completely insulated from the effects of a recession, program officials should take the likelihood of a recession into account in making job-training decisions.

Two options often suggested to improve the employment of the disabled are an expanded public employment program and a quota requirement for private firms.[12] Before a full-scale public employment drive for the disabled gets underway, it is wise to inquire whether every effort has been made to solve the problem through the private sector. The private sector can be encouraged and or even required to take reasonable action to place the disabled in jobs. Setting specific quantitative quotas may not be the most efficient solution particularly in light of the experience of other countries; perhaps it needs to be stated that for some portion of the disabled population, employment is not feasible and the best that can be hoped for is an adequate transfer payment and training in independent living skills.

An alternative to direct labor market intervention is the promulgation of laws establishing the rights of the handicapped and the responsibilities of firms in respect to hiring the handicapped. Two components of Title V of the Rehabilitation Act of 1973 were devoted to just such a purpose. Section 503 requires firms receiving government funds to undertake affirmative action in hiring the handicapped.[13] Section 504 requires nondiscriminatory behavior toward the handicapped. The recent origin of these sections leaves their ultimate value unclear.[14] Nonetheless as complaint procedures are improved and as disabled people and rehabilitation counselors become more familiar with the intricacies of the legislation, one could expect it to have far-reaching consequences. Together with the other labor market alternatives these laws can mean the difference between a job and welfare for a great many disabled people. The workings of the laws should be watched carefully, and failings should be corrected so that the true intent of the legislation can be fulfilled.

The Disabled and Their Activities

The final factor likely to affect the shape and success of rehabilitation in the future is the disabled themselves. The 1973 Rehabilitation Act stressed that priority be afforded the severely disabled. The result of this emphasis appears to have been a decreasing effectiveness in the state-federal rehabilitation program, at least in terms of rehabilitations. Yet the increasing concern about the equity with which public funds are allocated suggests that certain losses in efficiency are acceptable.

Predicting what the make-up of the severely disabled population will be in the future is a complicated task, but certain tendencies seem evident. For example, legal decisions stressing the rights of the mentally ill and the mentally retarded are sure to force more states to deemphasize institutional care, thereby increasing demand for such noninstitutional services as vocational rehabilitation.[15] Another change may be related to legalization and greater social acceptance of abortion as well as an improved capacity to detect malformed fetuses at early stages of development. The net effect of these two developments may mean a reduced population of persons disabled since childhood. Other medical improvements will lead to more of some impairments through life-saving efforts while other improvements could reduce certain impairments. It is this kind of knowledge that is central to a well-planned rehabilitation program.

As cited earlier, legislative initiatives have been quite extensive in recent years. A large part of the explanation for those actions can be found in the increasingly vocal and politically active disability organizations.[16] These advocacy organizations are certain to increase in the future both in size and in influence. While these developments may have their origin in other types of minority rights movements the disabled now appear to be breaking out on their own quite effectively. As for the impact on individual rehabilitation, it will probably be felt most through demands for accountability. In part, this is what the requirement for an individualized written rehabilitation plan is all about. In the future, rather than concentrate on what objectives are being pursued, advocates will more than likely start to pay more attention to what is achieved.

Along with demands for improved services, these organizations will surely lead the call for higher levels of cash transfers to support those disabled persons unable to return to work. Unfortunately no neat dividing line exists between those able and those unable to go back to work. As a result, some impaired individuals face a choice between working and not working. Anytime such a choice is feasible, the presence of a cash transfer will enhance the no work alternative. Thus the question is not whether there should be disincentives, but their size. Obviously the greater the disincentive the more difficult is the job of rehabilitation. Yet all the disabled should not be forced to accept something less than subsistence simply to spur on that portion of the disabled population that can return to work. The pendulum will probably swing back and forth as to what constitutes an acceptable degree of disincentives. For the near term, it seems that the pressure is greatest from those seeking to control spending and encourage employment. A reduced growth in real cash benefits may be in the offing. The result will likely be twofold: greater numbers of people will not apply for benefits in the first place and more recipients will demand rehabilitation services.

There is no certainty attached to these predictions just as there are no numbers to be precisely estimated. The magnitude of the disincentives built into the current system have never been accurately quantified. Furthermore the strength of the forces on the pendulum will depend on matters outside the disability policy arena. In particular, the condition of the economy may be the ultimate arbiter when it comes to fiscal matters in rehabilitation. The cyclical nature of the economy suggests constantly moving forces acting on rehabilitation. Perhaps the best that can be done is to try to predict the fluctuations and minimize the movement around some socially acceptable point.

In summation, the evidence in the rehabilitation field overwhelmingly documents the extreme complexity that faces policy makers. The task of meeting these challenges is a difficult one. It cannot and should not become a matter of making continued incremental legislative and programmatic changes after an event has occurred. We need to do a better job of predicting the future and preparing for it. It is with this objective in mind that the chapters in this volume were prepared. While it could be melodramatic to suggest that rehabilitation is at a crossroads, it is not incorrect to suggest that the 1980s will bring with them great demands for change in rehabilitation. Now is the time to prepare to meet those demands.

AN OVERVIEW

All the questions one might wish to ask about rehabilitation could not possibly be resolved in a single volume. In structuring the book, our general objective was to present a variety of perspectives on the performance of rehabilitation programs. Partly because rehabilitation is so closely connected with employment, the measurable outcome of success has often been judged in economic terms. An improved understanding of the economics of vocational rehabilitation can go a long way toward improving social policy decision making. These improvements are being demanded by legislators facing increasing pressure to trim public spending.

But although the economic theme runs through the entire volume, other aspects of rehabilitation are not neglected. In order to assure a wide range of methods and viewpoints, we chose contributors from several disciplines besides economics. Among those presenting their views are persons with backgrounds in social work, sociology, and rehabilitation administration.

The first chapter by Monroe Berkowitz, Martin Horning, Stephen McConnell, Jeffrey Rubin, and John D. Worrall, summarizes an economic analysis of the Beneficiary Rehabilitation Program (BRP) for DI recipients.

The usefulness of evaluations of rehabilitation programs is

well established. One tool in particular, benefit-cost analysis, has proven valuable in judging the success of rehabilitation efforts. But benefit-cost analysis is fraught with technical and data problems. The authors attempt to clarify these issues as they relate to evaluations of the BRP. The results of a new benefit-cost study are reported and provide some support for continued use of DI trust fund dollars for rehabilitation.

Even though the program has demonstrated its effectiveness flaws remain, particularly in financing and client selection. The authors consider ways to improve the decisions about total dollars available to rehabilitation and the allotment of those dollars to the states. They present some detailed suggestions for financing reforms designed to improve program performance.

Other policy actions to improve performance are considered in light of a multiple regression analysis that relates individual characteristics to the probability of termination of DI benefits due to employment. In addition, reforms of the DI program's benefit structure and regulations are discussed in light of the possibility that some existing rules pose a disincentive to terminate.

In Chapter 2, Sar Levitan and Robert Taggart argue that labor market realities make it necessary to reevaluate the goals and service priorities of the vocational rehabilitation system. Traditionally, the system has placed considerable emphasis on medical restoration of the disabled and on such nonvocational forms of assistance as counseling and social services. But the authors dispute the wisdom of such policies in a period when limited funds are available for rehabilitation and when the demand for labor is weak. They urge that a more realistic strategy would be to concentrate rehabilitation efforts on the improvement of client employability and on the generation of jobs.

Behind the authors' emphasis on job placement is a belief that vocational rehabilitation has not entirely succeeded as an employment and training program. Levitan and Taggart are critical of the benefit-cost analyses that have purported to demonstrate the program's effectiveness, and they recommend that the program be brought into line with the performance standards, as well as the policies, of other manpower programs.

In Chapter 3, the character of the "client experience" under the vocational rehabilitation program is examined by Marvin B. Sussman, a pioneer in sociologic analysis of rehabilitation. Sussman points to problems in the human service system as a whole and to certain contradictions in our policy toward the severely disabled, which have prevented many eligible persons from seeking or receiving services. He offers a sympathetic account of the growth of the client assertiveness movement, and identifies as the goals of this movement professional accountability, contractual treatment, and entitlement to services. He assigns particular importance to the efforts of client activists to challenge the assumptions that underlie the conventional model of patient-practitioner relations.

Sussman's own policy recommendations concern the role of the family in rehabilitation treatment. Noting that the family and friends of the disabled individual usually share in the economic and psychological consequences of disability, and that they may withhold or provide important supports to the individual, Sussman urges that rehabilitation strategies be designed that would permit family members and intimates a larger role in the rehabilitation process.

John Noble reports in Chapter 4 on his firsthand study of the foreign experience in rehabilitation. He documents the similar patterns across nations in the growth of the costs and incidence of disability. Two areas in particular are singled out for attention: The impact of improved medical care and the trend toward automation of the production process. The implications of automatic indexing of benefits are noted as is the lack of success a few countries have had in limiting such benefit increments.

The net effect of a growing disabled population at a time when job markets are weak has led several foreign nations to turn to created work in either a workshop environment or in the public sector. The attempts to improve rehabilitation through quotas, penalties, subsidies, and changes in the retirement age are also reviewed. In studying these programs, Noble was able to identify fourteen direct and indirect variables influencing rehabilitation outcomes. Each variable is discussed in light of the author's observation of the way they have affected rehabilitation performance.

On the basis of his international perspective, Noble seeks to draw some conclusions for the future of U.S. policy. His analysis implies a belief that the path being followed in the United States has already been traveled by some European nations. In light of the persistent problems plaguing these countries, one is left with strong doubts about future disability policy in the United States. The lessons from the foreign experience, Noble implies, will go unheeded.

In Chapter 5, George Welch, president of International Rehabilitation Associates, presents an argument for greater involvement of the private sector in rehabilitation. He asserts that the rehabilitation program that the private sector now offers has certain advantages including the prompt initiation of treatment, personalized attention, and expert vocational placement services. Rehabilitation personnel in the private sector are more knowledgeable about the business community than their public sector counterparts, and they understand the necessity of fitting their clients' marketable skills to available job opportunities. Welch also discusses how the factors of competition and accountability at play in the private sector contribute to more efficient and responsible services.

The last portion of the chapter treats the uneasy coexistence of the state/federal vocational rehabilitation program and the private rehabilitation programs at the present time. Welch identifies some of the issues which complicate the relationship of the two sectors, and calls for greater cooperation between them.

In Chapter 6, Donald Galvin, former director of the Michigan vocational rehabilitation agency, examines the effect of the 1973 Rehabilitation Act on administration at the state agency level. Pointing to the marked reduction in the number of successful rehabilitants since the passage of the Act gave priority to the severely disabled, Galvin suggests that state agencies lack both the experience and the resources to meet the comprehensive needs of this group. Galvin also discusses the predicament of the state vocational rehabilitation counselor under the legislation: Presented with a legislatively mandated change in the program's target population, counselors have had to administer a set of eligibility criteria that contain certain disincentives to the admission of severely disabled clients, in the face of continuing resistance by the labor market to the severely disabled worker.

In addition, Galvin looks at the impact of the Rehabilitation Act on the interagency network which makes up the entire rehabilitation system. He cites as two positive developments the efforts of state education, rehabilitation and social service agencies to design and implement joint programs, and the emergence of the Centers for Independent Living as significant new "colleagues" in the rehabilitation area. Galvin closes with recommendations concerning the refinement of federal program standards for service evaluation, and the development of a new index of successful case closure.

These chapters written by academics, practitioners, and long-time observers of the rehabilitation scene are testimony to the complexity of current problems faced by the rehabilitation program. The authors employ various methods of analysis, each of which is designed to shed light on the rehabilitation process. Some of the chapters are based on empirical analysis of the rehabilitation experience, whether in the general program or in a specialized program such as the one designed to rehabilitate Social Security DI recipients. Other authors depend on insights gained from administrative experience in rehabilitation agencies or from the experience of related manpower and social welfare programs.

The rehabilitation program in the United States has never stood still. Ever since its beginnings in the first quarter of this century it has exhibited remarkable flexibility. It has had to accommodate a changing clientele, changing rehabilitation methods, and of course, the changing expectations of Congress and the public. The challenges that it has faced in the past were probably easier to meet than the challenges, and perhaps the opportunities, posed by recent legislative amendments and changing consumer demands. For the programs to continue to prosper and meet these new challenges it is necessary to periodically reexamine the functioning of the program and the policy options that are best suited to program goals. The authors, each of them from his own perspective, contribute essential ingredients designed to help in meeting that challenge.

NOTES

1. For a discussion of the origins of today's disability policy see Edward Berkowitz, "The American Disability System in Historical Perspective," in E. Berkowitz (ed.), *Disability Policies and Government Programs* (New York: Praeger, 1979), and C. Esco Obermann, *A History of Vocational Rehabilitation in America* (Minneapolis: Denison, 1965).

2. Many of the issues surrounding disincentives in welfare programs are discussed in the context of an evaluation of President Carter's welfare reform proposal in *The Administration's Welfare Reform Proposal: An Analysis of the Program for Better Jobs and Income*, Budget Issue Paper for Fiscal Year 1979, Congressional Budget Office, Washington, D.C., April 1978.

3. The problems of the long term care sector are examined in Valerie LaPorte and Jeffrey Rubin (eds.), *Reform and Regulation in Long Term Care* (New York: Praeger, 1979).

4. The extent of poverty after transfer payments and the lack of health insurance are surveyed in two Congressional Budget Office Background Papers: *Welfare Reform: Issues, Objectives, and Approaches*, July 1977, and *Profile of Health Care Coverage: The Haves and Have-Nots*, March 1979.

5. An example of the application of cost-benefit analysis to rehabilitation is found in John D. Worrall, "A Benefit-Cost Analysis of the Vocational Rehabilitation Program," *Journal of Human Resources*, Vol. 13, No. 2 (Spring 1978), pp. 285–298.

6. See Saad Z. Nagi and Lawrence L. Riley, "Coping with Economic Crisis: The Disabled on Public Assistance," *Journal of Health and Human Behavior*, Vol. 9 (December 1968), pp. 317–327.

7. See Monroe Berkowitz, William G. Johnson, and Edward H. Murphy, *Public Policy Toward Disability* (New York: Praeger, 1976), Chapter 8, for an empirical assessment of the impact of disability benefits on the probability someone will apply for benefits.
8. Public employment is a key element in President Carter's welfare reform proposal. For an analysis of several strategies to increase employment generally see, John L. Palmer (ed.), *Creating Jobs: Public Employment Programs and Wage Subsidies* (Washington, D.C.: Brookings Institution, 1978).
9. A review and evaluation of the rehabilitation research field through the early 1970s can be found in Monroe Berkowitz, Valerie Englander, Jeffrey Rubin, and John D. Worrall, *An Evaluation of Policy-Related Rehabilitation Research* (New York: Praeger, 1975).
10. See Robert Counts (ed.), *Independent Living Rehabilitation for Severely Handicapped People: A Preliminary Appraisal* (Washington, D.C.: The Urban Institute, 1978).
11. See Joseph LaRocca and Jerry Turem, *The Application of Technological Development to Physically Disabled People* (Washington, D.C.: The Urban Institute, 1978), and Janet Brown and Martha Redden, *A Research Agenda on Science and Technology for the Handicapped*, Office of Opportunities in Science, American Association for the Advancement of Science, Washington, D.C., 1979.
12. A variety of employment strategies for the disabled are considered in the context of policy in Great Britain by Jack Wiseman and John Cullis, "Social Policy Towards Disabled Workers," in A. J. Culyer (ed.), *Economic Policies and Social Goals* (London: Martin Robertson, 1974).
13. Note that the legislation has a distinct definition of this group; it is not necessarily the same people we refer to as the disabled. For a clarification of these definitional issues see See Saad Z. Nagi, "The Concept and Measurement of Disability," in Edward Berkowitz, (ed.) *Disability Policies and Government Programs*.
14. See DePaul Law Review, *Symposium on Employment Rights of the Handicapped*, Vol. 27, No. 4 (Summer 1978).
15. For an analysis of the economic ramifications of the litigation see Jeffrey Rubin, *Economics, Mental Health, and the Law* (Lexington, Mass.: D.C. Heath, 1978).
16. The nature of this advocacy movement is explored in Frank Bowe, *Handicapping America: Barriers to Disabled People* (New York: Harper and Row, 1978).

Chapter 1

AN ECONOMIC EVALUATION OF THE BENEFICIARY REHABILITATION PROGRAM

**Monroe Berkowitz,
Martin Horning,
Stephen McConnell,
Jeffrey Rubin,
and John D. Worrall**

Since its inception some twenty-four years ago, the disability insurance (DI) component of the Social Security program has expanded rapidly. Concern for the DI program has grown of late in part because of the well publicized financial problems facing the Social Security System. Until passage of the Social Security Amendments of 1977, the solvency of the DI trust fund was in question. Solutions to a continuing excess of payments over receipts include raising taxes through rate increases and adjustments to the maximum taxable limit as well as reducing expenditures. A reduction in spending can come about either through lower benefits or fewer recipients.

In this chapter, we will explore the effectiveness of one effort, the Beneficiary Rehabilitation Program (BRP), to reduce the number of eligible recipients. Although an alternative approach, such as tightening the definition of disability, could achieve a similar reduction, the trend has been toward easing eligibility requirements. Furthermore, a program such as the BRP has the socially redeeming objective of seeking to return a disabled person to the workforce. The BRP attacks the problem of disability instead of avoiding it.

In the first section we will review the origin of the BRP, its method of operation, and some of the statistical evidence on the program's growth over time. In addition, methodology and the findings of a number of benefit-cost analyses of the BRP are critically examined. A more up-to-date benefit-cost study is reported and an assessment of program performance is made. The third section includes a review of how such evaluation criteria as efficiency, equity, and administrative convenience could be applied to alternative financing arrangements for the BRP. We then proceed to present and evaluate several alternative financing plans and develop a new method to determine total BRP spending as well as allotments of this total to the states. The fourth section of the chapter is devoted to an examination of the characteristics of those BRP clients who are successful enough in the labor market to allow them to leave the DI rolls. A regression model is used to measure the impact of a number of variables on the probability of termination. The evidence indicates that factors in the DI program may retard the success of the BRP. We close the chapter by considering reforms in the DI program designed to reduce the disincentives to return to work. (A postscript has been added to report on recent legislative and administrative changes.)

The BRP functions in a complex environment with changing DI benefit levels, changing objectives of the rehabilitation program and fluctuating labor market demand all influencing its performance. Dissatisfaction with its record has evoked calls for its discontinuation. Although our research would not support such drastic action, the results do suggest that complacency is inappropriate. And while more research would be helpful, our analysis indicates there is enough information for policy makers to begin the necessary reform of the BRP.

An Overview of the BRP

The Provisions and Purposes of the BRP

Social Security Disability Insurance Program. The SSDI program provides transfer payments to covered workers, and certain widows, widowers, and children of covered workers. To receive a payment, a beneficiary must have a physical or mental impairment that has lasted or is expected to last 12 months. The impairment must be of such severity as to prevent substantial gainful activity.

The DI program is financed through a payroll tax and is the largest single federal transfer program for the disabled. The number of people receiving benefits has risen rapidly over the last decade, as has the level of disbursements; and for a time, expenditures were exceeding receipts. Although the number of people on the DI rolls has increased rapidly, the number of people who have recovered and been removed from the rolls has not kept pace.

The Development of the BRP. When the legislation establishing the disability insurance program was drawn up, Congress emphasized that rehabilitation would be an important component of the new program.[1] Between 1954 and 1965, legislative amendments provided both a carrot and a stick to foster rehabilitation. In 1954, when an earnings freeze for disabled workers was passed, the law required the referral of disabled workers to state vocational rehabilitation agencies. When cash benefits were introduced in 1956, a similar referral provision was included, with the additional specification that benefits could be withheld or reduced if the disabled beneficiary refused rehabilitation services without good cause. In subsequent years, positive inducements were provided to encourage the beneficiary to return to work, if only for a short time. The creation of a trial work period protected those who sought active employment against the possibility of a permanent loss of benefits. Similarly, the elimination of the waiting period in cases of recurring disability meant that individuals who were unable to continue in a job could expect immediate restoration of benefits when they reentered the program.

Despite the rehabilitation requirements and the trial work provisions, however, the number of disability insurance beneficiaries receiving rehabilitation services remained small during the 1955–1965 period. Of the more than 2 million severely disabled persons receiving benefits, only about 19,000, or less than one percent, were rehabilitated by the state vocational rehabilitation agencies.[2] Over the same period only 1.9 percent of the total number of rehabilitated clients were disability beneficiaries.[3]

To improve agency performance in rehabilitating beneficiaries, Congress established the BRP as part of the 1965 Social Security Amendments. Because some states were having difficulty in matching the federal funding for the general vocational rehabilitation program, Congress provided DI trust fund money as 100 percent reimbursement to states for the cost of rehabilitation services to disabled beneficiaries. One obvious purpose of the amendments was to stimulate the state agencies to provide more vocational rehabilitation services to disability beneficiaries who had largely been neglected by the general rehabilitation program.

The objective of the BRP, however, was not only the provision of more services to more people, but also the restoration of the client to substantial gainful activity. The rationale for using trust funds to finance rehabilitation services was that 100 percent federal funding would be instrumental in removing persons from the DI beneficiary rolls and would, therefore, result in long-term savings to the trust fund.[4]

The Secretary of HEW was empowered to formulate criteria for the selection of individuals to receive BRP services based upon the effect the provision of services would have upon the trust fund.[5] As a result, four eligibility criteria were established as necessary for a beneficiary is to qualify for trust fund financing:

1. The disabling physical or mental impairment is not so rapidly progressive as to outrun the effect of vocational rehabilitation services or to preclude restoration of the beneficiary to productive activity.
2. The disability without the service planned is expected to remain at a level of severity resulting in the continuing payment of disability benefits.
3. A reasonable expectation exists that providing such services will result in restoring the individual to productive activity.
4. The predictable period of productive work is long enough that the benefits which would be saved and the contributions which would be paid to the trust funds from future earnings would offset the costs of planned service.[6]

Those beneficiaries who fail to meet the eligibility criteria for BRP services may, of course, still be eligible to receive services in the general vocational rehabilitation program.

Selection Procedures. The BRP is jointly administered by the Social Security Administration and the Rehabilitation Service Administration (RSA). The Rehabilitation Services Administration provides the client services and has operational responsibility. The Social Security Administration has responsibility for planning and evaluation, and for setting program policies and standards.

Admission to the BRP program begins with a referral from a Disability Determination Services (DDS) unit. The DDS unit in each state is responsible for selecting those applicants who are entitled to disability benefits. At the time of disability determination, the units also carry out a rough screening of applicants to identify those who may have vocational potential. If unit personnel believe that an applicant would be eligible for the BRP program or for rehabilitation services under the basic program, they fill out a referral form and send it, possibly with some of the medical evidence and a record of the district office interview, to the vocational rehabilitation agency. When the vocational rehabilitation agency receives the referral, it evaluates the applicant once again to determine whether he or she will be admitted to the general federal-state vocational rehabilitation program. Once the agency has completed its evaluation, it may then proceed to apply the special selection criteria described above in order to single out those applicants who are eligible for services under the BRP.

Clients accepted into either the BRP or the basic federal-state program are provided a variety of services designed to assist them in meeting their vocational goals. A rehabilitation counselor and beneficiary will draw up an individualized written rehabilitation plan that they will use as a guide toward rehabilitation. The services that are necessary to complete the individualized written rehabilitation plan and to accomplish the vocational goal may be provided by the rehabilitation agency or they may be purchased from other providers.

Closure and Goals. The goal of beneficiaries accepted into the basic federal-state program may be competitive employment, placement in a nonwage position such as homemaker or unpaid family worker, or employment in sheltered workshops. The goals for beneficiaries accepted into the BRP must be competitive employment *and* termination from the DI rolls. Rehabilitation is a necessary, but not a sufficient, condition for termination. To be rehabilitated, a beneficiary must be placed in competitive employment for a minimum of 60 days, but to be terminated, he must have left the DI rolls altogether.

Financing the BRP. The Senate Report on the Social Security Amendments of 1965 maintained that most states fell short of matching federal funds available for vocational rehabilitation and that the resulting insufficiency of funds constituted a substantial obstacle to the rehabilitation of a greater number of Social Security disability beneficiaries:

> Under present conditions, the States are not able to provide services for all handicapped people who apply and can benefit from them. It is natural that they give priority to applicants for such services who have the best rehabilitation potential. Social Security disability beneficiaries who are likely to be older and more severely disabled than other applicants for vocational rehabilitation, generally do not represent the best investment of the State's rehabilitation resources, and they often have a lower priority than others applying for rehabilitation services.[7]

These observations were probably more applicable in 1965 than they are at present. In the three-year period after 1962, the expenditures of the joint federal-state vocational rehabilitation program passed the $100 million mark and reached $154 million. At that time, the federal government provided 61.4 percent of the funding. By contrast, expenditures at the present time are close to $1 billion, and the federal government supplied 80 percent of the funds. The more generous federal matching of funds in the present program means that the 100 percent financing of the BRP is not, marginally, as attractive as it was when the federal government supplied only a little over half the funds for the general program. At the time of the 1965 amendments, the funding arrangements of the BRP provided a welcome source of funds that required no state matching. Today, with 80 percent federal matching, the differential is not as great. Nevertheless, the BRP continues to provide an additional source of monies to finance rehabilitation services. States consistently manage to spend a high percentage of their allotments under the BRP funding scheme, and the number of clients served has increased with expenditures.

At present, the BRP is financed by allotments that are drawn from the trust fund and allocated to each state in advance on a quarterly basis. The maximum amount of funds available for the program is a fixed amount of the previous year's Social Security DI payments. The proportion of the total allotment that each state receives is based upon the ratio of the number of beneficiaries residing within a given state to the total DI population.[8] A qualification alters slightly the distribution of funds derived from this formula: the allotment shall not be less than $150,000 to any state, nor less than $25,000 to any territory. If any distributional changes are necessary to comply with this condition, they are derived by proportionately reducing the allotments to each of the remaining states and territories.

Although the initial allotment to each state is independent of any measurement of performance, the final grant received by the state depends upon the amount of services provided to DI beneficiaries. The RSA uses a system of quarterly reporting by the states to estimate which states will run out of funds and which states will have a surplus. On the basis of these calculations, funds are redistributed in the latter part of the fiscal year in favor of those states that are more likely to use up their initial allotment.

Two Views on The Purpose of the BRP. Interviews with persons in RSA and the Social Security Administration indicate that the intent of Congress in passing the 1965 amendments has been variously interpreted. Some individuals stress the desire on the part of Congress to extend rehabilitation opportunities to a neglected group. The provision of 100 percent financing for eligible DI beneficiaries was designed to induce the agencies to provide effective rehabilitation services for a group whose members are, by definition, severely disabled. At a time when general funds had to be matched 40 cents on the dollar, BRP funds were available without any matching.

Moreover, in 1965 the severely handicapped did not enjoy the priority they were to be accorded by the Rehabilitation Act of 1973. The more generous financial arrangements and, as important, the actual dollar increase in funds, encouraged the state agencies to include DI beneficiaries as one of the client groups. Hence, many of those interviewed felt that the amendments were primarily intended to establish the necessary incentives so that the state agencies would serve DI beneficiaries and bring to this group the advantages of increased well-being that accompany rehabilitation.

The assumption underlying the views of these individuals is that savings to the trust fund are an incidental constraint, while the heart of the BRP is service to the person on the beneficiary rolls. Other individuals, however, including those who are charged with administering the BRP, bring a very different interpretation to the 1965 amendments. They stress that the DI trust fund is primarily a vehicle for wage replacement, designed to provide cash benefits to covered persons who suffer an impairment that prevents any substantial gainful employment. One must be cautious when diverting part of these funds for purposes other than the payment of benefits. This position leads them to argue that Congress is justified in such diversion only if it has the expectation that the size of the fund will not suffer in the long run. In support of their view, this group notes that the legislative amendments specify that savings are to result to the fund. While they concede that the amendments also speak of rehabilitating the "maximum number" of beneficiaries, they claim that the drafters of the amendment were acting on the assumption that a maximum number of rehabilitants would mean greater savings to the fund.

At the moment, we need not choose between these two views, nor should we reconcile them to some middle position that might destroy the essential insights of both. We can conclude from our brief examination of the development of the program that Congress did provide funds on a more generous basis than in the general program in order to provide services for a group they thought were underserved. It is also quite clear that the total program was to be operated so as to save the trust fund money in the long run.

In addition, it is apparent that conditions in the DI program and in the vocational rehabilitation program have changed since 1965. Severely handicapped persons are no longer strangers to the vocational rehabilitation agencies and the method of financing the general vocational rehabilitation programs now comes closer to 100 percent federal financing.

Statistical Trends of the BRP

Allotments and Expenditures. As we indicated earlier, the maximum amount of DI trust funds to be allocated among state agencies each year for the BRP is a fixed percentage of the year's total Social Security DI payments. Initially the percentage was 1 percent of total payments, but in response to an encouraging start by the program, the maximum was increased to 1.25 percent in 1973 and 1.50 percent in 1974.

Since 1972, however, the total amount of DI cash benefit payments increased rapidly from a little over $4 billion in mid-1972 to over $9 billion by mid-1976. The increase of almost 130 percent in DI benefit payments was a result of higher wages, an accelerating inflation rate, and legislative liberalization of benefit levels, as well as a substantial increase in beneficiaries. The number of beneficiaries in current payment status during the same period increased by 47 percent, from 3 million to 4.5 million.

The combined effect of the increased maximum limits (from 1 percent to 1.5 percent) and the accelerated growth of DI benefit payments resulted in an unanticipated increase in the amount of BRP funds available to the states. The allotment for fiscal year 1972 was $30.5 million, but by fiscal year 1976 the amount had reached $102.6 million, a staggering increase of over 230 percent in the dollar size of the program.[9]

In the DI program in general, taxes paid into the DI trust fund have not kept pace with the increased payment of benefits out of the trust fund. Consequently, the size of the DI trust fund has been diminishing, and there is every indication that it would have been exhausted by the end of 1979 if contribution rates and the maximum taxable income had not changed. We have noted already that the BRP allotments are based on a fixed percentage of benefit payments and not on a fixed percentage of the size of the trust fund. Because the increase in the size of the BRP allotments has coincided with the reduction in the trust fund size, the BRP has been taking an increasingly larger percentage of the trust fund. Even with the smaller allotments in 1977 and 1978 (less than the statutory 1.5 percent of benefits), the BRP's size has increased relative to that of the trust fund.[10]

Clients Served, Rehabilitations and Terminations

BRP expenditures have not only accounted for an increasingly larger percentage of the trust fund, but have also come to represent an increasingly larger share of the total expenditures on all vocational rehabilitation programs. In the first six years of operation, BRP expenditures averaged less than 4 percent of total vocational rehabilitation expenditures. Since 1972, the relative share has increased dramatically, reaching 9.2 percent in the fiscal year 1976.

Not surprisingly, the rapid growth of the BRP has raised questions about its effectiveness. Has the population served by the BRP expanded in such a way as to warrant the large growth in the funds allocated? Have beneficiaries been terminated from the rolls so as to produce savings to the trust fund?

Tables 1-1 and 1-2 present comparative statistics on the number of clients served and the number of rehabilitations for the BRP and the general program. The tables show that the increase in BRP expenditures has been matched by an increase in the number of clients served by the program, but not by the number of rehabilitations. The number of clients served per year has more than doubled since 1973, in keeping with the same proportional increase of expenditures. The number of rehabilitations per year increased more gradually to a peak of 13,358 in 1974 and then fell below 13,000 in 1975 and 1976. The BRP has, however, been serving and rehabilitating an increasingly larger percentage of the total number of clients served and rehabilitated by the vocational rehabilitation program over the last five years. The relative increase has been a result of the

Table 1-1 Number of Clients Served by State Vocational Rehabilitation Agencies by Type of Program

Fiscal Year	Unduplicated Count of Clients Served General Program*	BRP	BRP Count as a % of Total Count
1976	1,118,991	88,449	7.0
1975	1,143,155	75,667	6.0
1974	1,201,661	62,719	4.9
1973	1,136,646	39,799	3.4
1972	1,077,691	33,354	3.0
1971	971,784	29,876	3.0
1970	846,310	29,601	3.4

*Clients served under Section 110, 1974–1976 and under basic support program of Section 2, 1970–1973.

Source: Annual Reports of State Vocational Rehabilitation Agency Program Data, Department of Health, Education and Welfare, Washington, D.C., 1970–1976.

Table 1-2 Number of Rehabilitations Reported by State Vocational Rehabilitation Agencies by Type of Program

Fiscal Year	Number of Rehabilitations General Program*	BRP	BRP Rehabilitations as a % of Total
1976	283,906	12,826	4.2
1975	306,021	12,585	3.9
1974	345,288	13,358	3.7
1973	349,146	11,580	3.2
1972	316,155	9,983	3.1
1971	281,482	9,790	3.4
1970	257,668	9,307	3.5
1969	233,392	7,998	3.3
1968	202,018	5,900	2.8

*Rehabilitations under Section 110, 1974–1976 and under basic support program of Section 2, 1968–1973.

Source: Ralph Treitel, "Effect of Financing...," p. 19 and *Program Data* reports, 1974–1976.

decline in the numbers served and rehabilitated in the general program; a decline which was influenced by the Rehabilitation Act of 1973 and the consequent emphasis on the rehabilitation of the severely disabled in the general program.

One final statistical trend which the analyst must consider is the average cost per rehabilitation in the general program and the BRP. The evidence indicates that the costs of rehabilitating a client are higher under the BRP than in the general program. For example, in 1976 the cost per rehabilitation in the general program was $3,161 while in the BRP it was $7,500. Such a difference is to be expected; more surprising, however, is the rapid rate of increase in the costs of rehabilitation under the BRP, relative to the rate of increase under the general program: 14 percent between 1973 and 1974, as compared with 12 percent in the general program; 52 percent beween 1974 and 1975, as compared with 21 percent in the general program; and 16.5 percent between 1975 and 1976, as compared with 11 percent in the general program.

The general conclusion to be drawn from Tables 1-1 and 1-2 and from the evidence concerning average rehabilitation costs is that BRP expenditures over the last few years have increased in almost direct proportion to the increase in the number of clients served. The increase in expenditures has not produced, however, a comparable change in the number of rehabilitations, and as a result, the cost per rehabilitation has been rising rapidly.

We have seen also that the BRP expenditures have claimed an increasing percentage of the total assets of the DI trust fund at the same time as the trust fund, for other reasons, has diminished. As a result, there is renewed interest in the effectiveness of the BRP. Particular attention is being paid to the relationship between expenditures and the eventual savings to the trust fund brought about by termination of the BRP client from the DI beneficiary rolls. In the next section, we will examine previous benefit-cost studies of the program and calculate a revised estimate of our own.

The Impact of the BRP on the DI Trust Fund

In this section, we present an estimate of the benefits and costs of the BRP with respect to the DI Trust Fund. We compare the present discounted value of the savings that accrue to the trust fund as a result of the program with the cost of operating the program. Our analysis is very restricted in its aims, but we regard it as an appropriate test of the program's adherence to the legislative mandate. Before we begin our own analysis, however, we consider the findings of earlier benefit-cost studies.

Social Security Administration (SSA): The Office of the Actuary

The SSA has been charged with the responsibility of evaluating the efficiency of the BRP, and has periodically issued its findings and informed the Congress of the results. The first evaluation of the BRP appeared in a series of memoranda written by the SSA actuary.[11] The actuary pointed up some of the problems which would recur in later evaluations of the program. The author's main conclusion was that the program was not paying for itself, but he attributed this failure to the fact that the program was in its infancy and sufficient time had not elapsed to allow for the terminations that would eventually result. The "time lag" or "pipe-line" problem has continued to create problems for analysts of the program's efficiency.

Subsequent studies of the BRP have all reported benefit-cost ratios above 1. For example, in 1970, the Office of the Actuary estimated the benefit-cost ratio for the program through fiscal year 1970 as 1.60.[12] A memorandum to the Commissioner of Social Security[13] points out that this study did not include the amount of taxes that terminees would subsequently pay into the trust fund, nor a deduction for those terminees who would have relapsed and returned to the disability rolls with full restoration of benefits.

The Office of the Actuary reasoned that the benefits from

taxes exceeded the benefits lost from relapse, given a 5 percent rate of relapse. Consequently, the actuary's estimated benefit-cost ratio was conservative. They also wanted to avoid wage projections that required assumptions as to unemployment, income levels, and relapse rates. In addition, they realized that insufficient time had elapsed since the beginning of the program to allow them to place great confidence in any one relapse rate.

In January 1972, another SSA estimate was released which covered the program through fiscal year 1971.[14] Using the same basic methodology as the earlier studies, the SSA reported a benefit-cost ratio of 1.93.

Committee Staff Report on the Disability Insurance Program, 1974

More recently, in a Committee Staff Report for the Committee on Ways and Means of the U.S. House of Representatives, the SSA Office of the Actuary reported the benefit-cost ratio of the program at 2.50 for terminations through fiscal year 1973.[15] Among the assumptions used in the study were an interest rate of 6 percent and a rate of inflation of 3 percent. The authors also assumed the PIA (Primary Insurance Amount) was a good proxy for the individual worker's benefit. The benefit streams were reduced by the ultimate termination rates from the program period, 1957–1968. These ultimate termination rates contained an adjustment for both mortality and medical recovery. A final assumption was that the inclusion of a computation for tax payback of the recovered cases would have offset any adjustments for recidivism and raised the reported benefit-cost ratio.[16]

Of necessity, the assumptions on inflation and interest rates are arbitrary. The SSA selected 6 percent as the discount rate, because the long-term bond rate was generally believed to be the best proxy for the long-term interest rate. Interest rates have gone above the 6 percent figure and unless the long-term trend brings them down, the choice of 6 percent would overestimate the benefits attributable to the program.

The choice of a 3-percent inflation rate could result in an underestimate of program savings. If actual inflation rates continue to stay high, the bias created will tend to counter bias due to the choice of the interest rate.

The adjustment for mortality or recovery — ultimate termination — based upon program experience for the period 1957–1968 should have little effect on the savings estimates. There was a more severe definition of disability during that period, but changes in ultimate termination rates have been marginal.

The PIA was used as a proxy for the individual worker's benefit. In order to calculate savings attributable to the program, the benefit that recovered workers would have received if they had remained on the rolls is compounded from the date of termination to age 64. The savings stream is adjusted for ultimate recovery and discounted.

Similarly, the benefits that would have been paid to other family members must be calculated. The time period for the compounding of these auxiliary savings is often less than it is for the primary beneficiary. The benefit for children will stop, for example, depending upon a child's age and education status, at age 18. A spouse's benefit status will depend upon the presence or absence of children. The Office of the Actuary makes adjustments to account for these facts; they do not, however, use separate mortality or recovery rates for other family members, although the absence of such refinements should not have a large effect on the benefit estimates.

Along with problems created by inconsistencies in the data files used, the 1974 study also contains some questionable methodological procedures. For example, no adjustment is made for recidivism. This decision, as we noted earlier, is based on the belief that tax payback of recoveries is larger than losses from recidivism.

A second source of error could arise from benefits being computed only for those terminated through FY 1973 while the costs are considered for the same period. There is a lag between the expenditure of trust funds for rehabilitation services and termination. Failing to adjust on either the benefit side or the cost side will understate the benefit-cost ratio.

There is also no consideration given to those rehabilitations financed with DI trust funds that never get reported to the SSA. The omission could result in an underestimate of the benefit-cost ratio of the program.

The General Accounting Office (GAO) Report

On May 13, 1976, the Comptroller General released the results of an independent study of the BRP and appended its policy recommendations.[17] The principal finding, that the benefit-cost ratio of the program was only 1.15, may have been influential in the decision to freeze and eventually reduce the level of program funding.

The GAO also used the computer program written by the Office of the Actuary to compute benefits attributable to the BRP. Consequently, they assumed a 6-percent interest rate, 3-percent inflation rate, and the 1957–1968 ultimate termination rates.

They did not compute tax payback nor make any adjustments for recidivism. The GAO Report does, however, claim that recidivism "was greater in fiscal year 1974 (2,228) than the total for the first seven years of the program (2,112).... If this increase in the recidivism rate continues, it could invalidate the SSA actuary's formula for computing savings."[18]

The GAO examined a sample of 350 beneficiaries from 4 states who had been rehabilitated and who had subsequently terminated from the DI rolls. The sample period was January 1971 to December 1973. They reported that 62 percent of their sample should not have had their terminations attributed to the BRP.[19] The claim was made that 51 percent of the sample did not meet the selection criteria for the program because they were scheduled for medical reexamination. In many cases the medical reexamination was seen by the GAO as strong evidence that there was an expectation of medical recovery. (Cases that are scheduled for medical reexamination are called "diaried cases.") In addition, GAO claimed that 11 percent of the terminated beneficiaries in its sample did not receive rehabilitation agency services.

There are several shortcomings in the GAO sample and in the subsequent determination of cases to be counted as contributors to trust fund savings. First, the sample is drawn from four states only. Since the selection process may differ widely from state to state, there is no guarantee that the GAO results are applicable nationwide.

Furthermore, the sample is based on an incomplete sampling frame. As we mentioned earlier, many rehabilitated beneficiaries are never reported to the SSA. Hence, when the benefits of cases GAO considers to be valid for inclusion in the benefit computation are expanded to estimate the population benefits, the expansion is done on the basis of an understated population.

The GAO examined cases inappropriately charged to the DI trust fund but did not examine cases inappropriately charged to the basic federal-state program. It can be legitimately claimed that their mandate was simply to estimate the benefit-cost ratio for cases receiving trust funding, but examining cases that should have been assigned to the DI trust fund would have provided some insight into the potential benefit-cost ratio.

The way in which the decision was made to assign cases as appropriate for inclusion or exclusion in the benefit calculation was not reported. The GAO has said that it was liberal in its assignment of cases, but it is not known if one investigator or ten decided how to assign individual cases, or if there was uniformity among investigators in the assignment of cases.

A Revised Estimate of Benefits and Costs in the BRP

The Data Base. The only data base available for our estimate of the benefit-cost ratio of the program is a computer tape of information recorded on the SSA 853 form. The tape has information on 56,040 beneficiaries who were rehabilitated by the BRP and reported to the SSA through December 1975. The 853 tape has only 69.7 percent of the number of rehabilitations reported in the RSA Quarterly Status Reports.

In his 1973 article Treitel attributes some of the difference to nonreceipt of form SSA-853 (Vocational Rehabilitation Report to SSA), and some data-processing problems. He also points out that until recently, all closure records were also matched with an administrative file consisting of earlier verification reports that the applicant for rehabilitation services was a disabled beneficiary. Incomplete matches resulted in much statistical data loss. Beneficiaries reported as rehabilitated, but not in competitive employment, were excluded from the statistical file in the past.

It is unfortunate that beneficiaries closed into noncompetitive employment had been excluded. Some of the rehabilitants may have subsequently moved to competitive employment and terminated as a result of their rehabilitation experience. Treitel makes a similar point regarding beneficiaries who were excluded from the file because they were not successfully rehabilitated. Treitel assumes that most of the trust fund rehabilitants omitted from the verified file were not disabled beneficiaries or not beneficiaries rehabilitated into competitive work capacity.

It is also quite possible that the underreporting problem is the result of keypunching errors, the failure to forward 853 Forms to SSA, and possibly the failure to consolidate into a single source the responsibility for insuring the timely receipt and processing of accurate data.

Other problems complicate the reliance upon a microdata file that was not designed as a tool for a benefit-cost study. One problem was that many individual records had no month of closure. Another problem was the thirteen percent (3,261 of 25,174) of the terminations we considered were closed as rehabilitated after they had terminated from the DI rolls. These and other problems with the data source indicate that one should be cautious in interpreting the results of the benefit-cost analysis.

Revised Estimate Methodology. For the purposes of deriving a benefit-cost estimate we used the same inflation rate (3 percent), discount rate (6 percent), and ultimate termination rates as those assumed by the Office of the Actuary and the GAO. We used the same computer program, with a minor revision, to compute the benefit payments that could be expected to be saved as a result of terminations generated by the BRP.

We included in our benefit computation those payments from the trust fund that were saved during the time that single and double recidivists were off the DI rolls. We also estimated the tax payback to the trust fund and attempted to deal with the pipeline problem. In order to account for some of the return on BRP expenditures made through FY 1973, we compared costs through FY 1973 with the benefits derived from all cases available on the 853 tape that were closed rehabilitated through calendar 1973 and subsequently terminated.

We selected all those cases with a rehabilitation closure year earlier than or equal to 1973. We also included those cases that had a termination year of 1973 or earlier, regardless of closure year. Our total number of terminations using these selection criteria was 15,079.

Benefit Calculation. We assumed that the PIA was a good proxy for the individual worker's benefit and that the maximum family benefit was a good proxy for the beneficiary's family benefit. In Table 1-3, we present our estimates, based on these assumptions of the benefit payments that were or will be saved by the trust fund as a result of the 15,079 terminations considered. The value, in constant 1966 dollars, of trust fund savings from this source is over $330 million. The average value of a termination to the trust fund has changed little over the period 1969 to 1975.

Table 1-3 Savings Through Terminations
(N = 15,079)

Fiscal Year	Number Terminated	Current Year Value of Savings	Present Value of Savings*	Present Value of Savings Per Termination in Constant 1966 Dollars
1967	199	$ 2,884,446	$ 2,721,194	$13,674
1968	984	19,189,808	17,078,861	17,356
1969	1,938	54,395,568	45,671,568	23,566
1970	2,243	61,310,768	48,563,871	21,651
1971	2,092	63,535,216	47,477,209	22,695
1972	2,367	79,970,554	56,376,078	23,818
1973	2,113	73,771,104	49,061,997	23,219
1974	1,884	65,596,672	41,156,164	21,845
1975	964	32,906,880	19,477,532	20,205
1976	295	5,353,953	2,989,619	10,134 [†]
			$330,574,093	

*The present value of savings represents the additional amount of money that would have had to be in the trust fund on July 1, 1966, in order to pay the additional benefits if the disabled beneficiaries had remained on the rolls and if interest accrued at 6 percent per year.

[†] This figure is not representative because we are only looking at people rehabilitated through 1973.

In light of the GAO's research on inappropriately assigned cases, we have also computed the savings to the trust fund based on the assumption that only 38 percent of the cases we considered were eligible (Table 1-4). We also assumed that 38 percent of the appropriately assigned cases would account for 39.7 percent of the total group savings.

Recidivism. It is not uncommon for a beneficiary to be rehabilitated and terminate, and then to relapse and return to the DI rolls. When we examined the history fields of those with a rehabilitation closure year earlier than or equal to 1973, we

Table 1-4 Termination Savings with GAO Assumptions in Closure Year 1973 or Earlier (N=15,079)

Fiscal Year	Number Terminated*	Current Year Value of Savings†	Present Value of Savings‡
1967	76	$ 1,145,125	$ 1,080,314
1968	374	7,618,354	6,780,308
1969	736	21,595,040	18,131,612
1970	852	24,340,375	19,279,857
1971	795	25,223,481	18,848,452
1972	899	31,748,306	22,381,303
1973	803	29,287,128	19,477,613
1974	715	26,041,879	16,338,997
1975	366	13,064,031	7,732,580
1976	112	2,125,519	1,186,879
			$131,237,915

*This is the number terminated *assuming* an ineligibility rate of 62 percent, the rate reported by the GAO in *Improvements Needed in Rehabilitating Social Security Disability Insurance Beneficiaries*, Department of Health, Education and Welfare, (MWD-76-66), May 13, 1976.

†This is the value of current year savings *assuming* that the 38 percent of terminations considered eligible by the GAO account for 39.7 percent of the total benefits. The 39.7 percent was derived from unpublished data provided by the GAO.

‡The present value of savings represents the additional amount of money that would have had to be in the trust fund on July 1, 1966, in order to pay the additional benefits if the disabled beneficiaries had remained on the rolls and if interest accrued at 6 percent per year.

found 3,585 cases that were recidivists. This recidivism count yields a recidivism rate (net) of 19.2 percent.

The figure of 3,585 recidivists includes 3,431 cases of single recidivism and 154 cases of double recidivism. In addition, our search of the history fields revealed that most recidivists return to the DI rolls in the first three or four years following termination.

In order to compute the payments that were saved during the time that recidivists were off the DI rolls, we used the individual worker's payments as recorded in the history field at the month of termination. We cumulated saved payments until the month of return to the DI rolls. The monthly payment amount was inflated by the actual benefit rate increase for each year that the beneficiary remained off the DI rolls.

To account for the fact that the family benefit is higher than the individual amount reported in the history field, we inflated the savings amount by a factor of 1.3. This factor is derived by assuming that the average family benefit for a beneficiary with a spouse and children is 1.6 times the individual benefit. Our research indicates that 39.5 percent of the terminated cases had no dependents. On the basis of these calculations, we estimate that approximately $13 million in constant 1966 dollars were saved during the period recidivists were off the DI rolls.

Benefit-Cost Ratios. If there were no further recidivism among terminated cases, and if we did not consider tax payback in our benefit calculation, the benefit-cost ratio of the program would be 1.17. It must be stressed that this figure is determined by assuming that 62 percent of the terminations were cases that had been assigned inappropriately. In addition, it is likely that the benefit stream is understated because there have been terminations that have occurred but have not been included on the 853 tape. Table 1-5 presents a summary of savings and costs with an assumption of no additional recidivism.

To refine the figures, we can adjust benefits downward for future recidivism in the following fashion. We will assume that anyone who terminated in FY 1972 or earlier will remain off the rolls. We will also assume that there will be an additional 100 percent recidivism in those cases terminated in FY 1973 or later. This would mean an additional 285 cases from 1973, an additional 152 cases from 1974, and an additional five cases from 1975. In the benefit stream we included only 38 percent of these 442 cases. We can deduct the savings for 108 cases in 1973, 58 cases in 1974, and 2 cases in 1975. Such an exercise reduces the benefit stream by $4 million and lowers the benefit-cost ratio to 1.14. One additional adjustment could be made to allow us to

Table 1-5 Present Value of Savings and Costs in Closure Year 1973 or Earlier

Fiscal Year	Present Value of Recidivist Savings*	Present Value of Termination Savings†	Total Savings Present Value	Present Value of Costs‡ (000)
1967	$ 48,873	$ 1,080,314	$ 1,129,187	$ 9,231
1968	208,844	6,780,308	6,989,152	14,231
1969	947,309	18,131,612	19,078,921	14,741
1970	$ 1,802,704	19,279,857	21,082,561	16,621
1971	2,315,680	18,848,452	21,164,132	18,215
1972	2,414,775	22,381,303	24,796,078	21,411
1973	2,410,462	19,477,613	21,888,075	28,552
1974	1,940,426	16,338,997	18,279,423	
1975	830,900	7,732,580	8,563,480	
1976	71,639	1,186,879	1,258,518	
	$13,456,937	$131,237,915	$144,694,852§	$123,502

*Assumes that all recidivists were eligible for the program.

†Assumes that 38 percent of the terminations were eligible and that they accounted for 39.7 percent of the benefits.

‡Includes $500,000 for 1966. The present value of costs represents the amount of money that would have had to be in the trust fund on July 1, 1966, in order to pay for the expenses incurred in the year of rehabilitation of disabled beneficiaries if the trust fund interest accrues at 6 percent per year.

§Includes $465, 325 for double termination.

understand the sensitivity of the results to GAO's claim that 62 percent of terminations were inappropriately assigned to the BRP.

Our research indicates that approximately 13 percent of the recidivists have subsequently reterminated and left the DI rolls. We could adjust benefits up for this phenomena, and use a more sophisticated technique to adjust benefits downward for recidivism, but the results would be marginal.

If we applied the RSA finding that the inappropriately assigned case rate is only 25 percent and assumed this rate held in the past, the benefit-cost ratio for the program would be 2.11.

Tax Payback. Although the amount of tax payback exceeds the deduction for recidivism, it has not been included in our benefit calculations. We have excluded payback because of the possibility that the taxes paid into the trust fund by a recovered worker could have been paid by another worker prior to the rehabilitant's return to work. In other words, we cannot assume that a terminee moves into a newly created job in the economy, rather than simply displacing another worker.

While discounting tax payback as a factor in our calculations, we have thought it advisable to reach an estimate of the payback to the DI trust fund. To calculate tax payback, we assumed a rate of wage increase of 5 percent, a discount rate of 6 percent, and an unemployment rate of 6 percent. To compute tax payback from termination year to 1974, we used the 1974 earnings level and assumed that earnings had grown at a rate of 5 percent since termination year.

To compute the tax payback from 1974 to age 64, we compounded 1974 earnings over time with a growth rate of 5 percent and a mortality adjustment. This admittedly crude procedure produced an estimate of $6 million (in 1966 dollars) that we could expect terminated workers to pay into the DI Trust fund. The joint employer-employee contribution would thus total $12 million.

Conclusions and Recommendations

Our revised estimate of the benefit-cost ratio for the BRP shows that, even with the assumptions of a high ineligibility rate and no tax payback, the program has had a benefit-cost ratio above 1. In addition, we suspect that our estimate of 1.17, although based on the best available data, understates the true value because records have been lost in the current data system.

It is obvious to anyone attempting these types of calculations that a data base suitable for evaluating the BRP should be developed as soon as possible. The responsibility for overseeing a management information system should be fixed clearly. Sampling procedures and cross validation checks need to be instituted to insure the accuracy of information in the system, and data should be included that cover both rehabilitated and nonrehabilitated cases.

Alternative Financing Schemes

One of the major recommendations in the GAO report was that the determination of the spending limit in the BRP be altered from its current fixed percentage method to a system whereby the amount allocated would be a direct function of the program's performance. The authors of the report proposed this change because the funds available for the BRP were growing rapidly, while the benefit-cost ratio appeared to be declining.

In responding to the GAO report, HEW agreed that the present fixed percentage method of funding was no longer appropriate. They undertook to "investigate alternative approaches to linking BRP funding to state agency performance and cost savings to the trust fund."

In this section, we examine some criteria by which a financing scheme can be evaluated. We then proceed to review several financing reform options in relation to these criteria and their impact on the amount allocated to individual states.

Evaluation Criteria

Several categories of tests can be used to evaluate the alternative financing plans. The tests we propose are the usual ones of efficiency and equity, and an additional one which, for want of a better term, we label administrative convenience. By efficiency, we mean technical efficiency: How well does a plan use funds to achieve the final goal of net savings to the trust fund? In the most efficient plan, given a limit on the size of the annual BRP appropriation, it would not be possible to shift one dollar of the trust fund appropriated for the BRP from one client to another or from one agency to another, and increase the net savings to the trust fund. If there were no limit on the annual BRP appropriation, we would have to add another condition: it would not be possible to increase the net savings by spending another dollar. We do not expect to implement such an ideal plan in the real world, but we can think of optimal efficiency as a criterion by which to judge individual financing plans in order to determine whether some are more efficient than others.

The test of equity or fairness brings into play a different set of considerations. We recognize a wide variety of notions about equity, some based on equal access to services, others on extent of disability or income position. Efficiency and equity considerations often conflict and as a result tradeoffs will be necessary.

Administrative convenience is a poor name for an important test. To be seriously considered by administrators, any plan must be based upon information the program can provide in time and in a manner that is useful for allotment purposes. Information about the outcomes of those served by the BRP is not immediately available. Any plan requires estimates or proxies for savings, and the ones chosen should meet the test of administrative convenience. They must be available in "real time" and without undue disruption to the administration of the BRP.

Efficiency.   The determination of an optimal amount of rehabilitation requires an understanding of the effects of increments of spending for vocational rehabilitation services on the probability of termination and eventual savings to the trust fund. In the ideal efficient system, sums will be expended for services until the last dollar spent on a client will result in a dollar of savings. If a single additional dollar were spent, it would yield less than a dollar in savings to the trust fund.

A hypothetical situation could exist where a counselor tries to plan his expenditures in light of these relationships. If he spends $100 on an evaluation measure and if that is all he spends, he is pretty confident that the client will not be closed rehabilitated, that the trust fund will be out $100, and that savings will be nil. If he spends an additional $100, he can spend more counseling time that, he reasons, will help the client's emotional stability, but will not greatly enhance his chance of successfully completing the program. A third $100 will buy the physical restoration services that are likely to result in the client's rehabilitation and that will give the client a good chance of termination. It is the counselor's best judgment that the termination will save the fund $1,000. But without more in the way of services, the counselor believes that the termination will be temporary and that the client will once again return to the rolls. Should he spend more?

In Table 1-6, we assume that the counselor can plan spending in these $100 increments, and that up to a point, with each increment he improves the quality of the rehabilitation and the probability that the client will stay off the rolls for a longer period of time. Given no constraints on funds, he should continue to spend on the client as long as each successive $100 increment yields marginal savings above $100. At line 6, he has spent a total of $600 and he expects total savings to the fund to be $9,000,

Table 1-6 Hypothetical Illustration of Costs and Savings for One Client

Line #	Marginal Cost of Rehab. Services	Total Cost of Rehab. Services	Total Savings to Trust Fund	Marginal Savings to Trust Fund	Net Savings to Trust Fund
1	$100	$ 100	0	0	−$100
2	100	200	0	0	− 200
3	100	300	$ 1,000	$1,000	700
4	100	400	3,000	2,000	2,600
5	100	500	6,000	3,000	5,500
6	100	600	9,000	3,000	8,400
7	100	700	10,000	1,000	9,300
8	100	800	10,100	100	9,300
9	100	900	10,100	0	9,200
10	100	1,000	10,100	0	9,100
11	100	1,100	10,100	0	9,000

and the crucial item — net savings, that is, the total savings minus the total costs — to be $8,400. An additional $100 expenditure (line 7) yields an additional $1,000 of savings for a net savings of $9,300. Increasing expenditures for services by another $100 raises total savings by $100 for a new total of $10,000, which, in our hypothetical example is the extent of the improvement that can be accomplished with respect to savings to the trust fund. Spending additional dollars on services yields no· additions to total savings. Nevertheless, the net savings, although declining, are positive and substantial.

For individual efficiency decisions, the framework just described is sufficient. With no constraint on total spending, no problem of client selection exists. All those who meet the eligibility criteria can be served so long as the marginal dollar expended is equal to the marginal benefit received and net savings to the fund are positive.

If there is some ceiling on appropriations, the problem is quite different. To make the discussion simpler, we can think of an agency faced with a group of potential DI beneficiary clients. Assume that we know, or can reasonably estimate, the cost of an efficient amount of rehabilitation for each client. Assume also that we have some good estimate of the savings to the fund. (The four special selection criteria require estimates of the same general character.) Thus, we have for each such individual an estimated cost, estimated savings, and a benefit-cost ratio, always narrowly defined in terms of savings to the fund and costs chargeable to the fund.

What is the most efficient way to allocate a fixed sum for services among the group? We cannot simply choose to serve first those with high individual benefit-cost ratios. The solution is to pick that combination of persons whose rehabilitations will result in the greatest aggregate net savings to the fund. No formula can assure that the correct combination is identified, but with knowledge of each person's benefits and costs the best combination can be selected.

If each state agency adopted the methodology described here as the basis of its selection procedure, allocations would not necessarily be efficient on a nationwide scale. If the allocations are based on some factor that is independent of net savings (for example, if they are based upon the number of beneficiaries, as in the present system) then the agencies may arrive at very different cut-off points. The last dollar spent in state A may yield a net savings of $1,000, whereas in state B the net savings might be $5,000. Under these conditions, the aggregate net savings to the fund would be increased if we shifted funds from A to B. State A would then rehabilitate fewer persons and state B more. The most efficient point would be reached where the marginal savings for the marginal dollar spent, or the ratio of marginal savings to marginal spending, is the same in each state.

Equity. It is important that clients of vocational rehabilitation agencies be treated fairly. To serve only those beneficiaries who show promise of termination, or to give the moderately disabled priority over the severely disabled in the provision of services, may violate equity criteria.

Congress did not specify any equity tests when it established the BRP. In the Rehabilitation Act of 1973, however, Congress directed the rehabilitation agencies to give priority to the severely handicapped. It might be difficult for any agency to arrange the order of preference for its general clients one way and to rank DI beneficiaries in another. It might be considered unfair to seek out the most severely handicapped among the applicants in the general program and then to "cream" the beneficiary population, taking cases easiest to rehabilitate first and those with lesser probability of rehabilitation and eventual termination next. Hence, in light of these equity considerations, we might propose a ranking of clients based upon the severity of their impairments. It would also be possible to rank clients according to their economic position; agencies could be directed in the interest of fairness or equity to give priority to those who are the poorest. A third possibility would be to grant services on a proportional basis for each type of disability. For example, under this arrangement, the number of services available to the blind would be based upon their relative numbers in the population.

The present allocation scheme does not link funding to performance, and consequently meets a type of equity criteria. Funds are allocated based upon the number of DI beneficiaries in each state. Thus, if financial considerations are the only constraints, all DI beneficiaries who meet the special selection criteria theoretically have an equal chance of receiving rehabilitation services regardless of the performance record of the state in which they reside.

Administrative Convenience. There is a third standard that is institutional in nature and that incorporates both efficiency and equity considerations. That third standard is based on what RSA refers to as the unique multiyear nature of rehabilitation services. Governments generally provide funding on a yearly basis; next year's funds are based on this year's data, or perhaps last year's data, and are generally guaranteed for one year only.

In order to meet standards of administrative convenience, a funding scheme would have to assure the agency that its year-to-year funding will not fluctuate erratically. It would relate levels of funding as closely as possible to current year's activities and recognize the cash flow problem of agencies.

Some Characteristics of Financing Plans

We have outlined the disagreement about the exact intent of Congress in passing the legislative provisions for the BRP. To some extent, one's interpretation of the congressional intent shapes one's views towards financing schemes. If the motive of Congress was to make services more readily available, then the interests of the provider agency might be given greater consideration. On the other hand, if the motive was to ensure savings to the trust fund, then payment should be made on the basis of results. Most of the schemes we describe are allotment plans that pay for services rendered, so that the real issue becomes whether funds are allotted on the basis of population factors, services rendered, or results. But for the moment let us recognize that the dichotomy between payment on the basis of services and payment on the basis of results can be exaggerated. Results, that is, terminations and consequent savings to the fund, are at the end of a road that begins with the acceptance of an eligible DI beneficiary as a client, and continues with the provision of services leading to the client's eventual rehabilitation.

The link between rehabilitations and terminations, however, can be a tenuous one. RSA points out:

> Terminations depend on too many unpredictable factors, including opportunities for employment and salary levels, which are generally governed by local and regional conditions and . . . disincentives to rehabilitation.[20]

Still, whether or not a person terminates is not wholly independent of the quality and type of his rehabilitation, and the quality of rehabilitation should, in turn, be related to the services provided.

In general, then, we can think of (1) plans that reward agencies for services performed and that do not allot any portion of the funds on the basis of results and (2) plans that reward on the basis of results without regard for services performed. The more confident we are of the closeness of the relationship between services and results, the more indifferent we will be as to the type of plan chosen. The thrust of the GAO report was to cast doubt on the closeness of the relationships and to reveal a preference for some plan that would be weighted more heavily in favor of payment on the basis of results. Our examination of historical trends has shown that increased funds have been used for increased services, without a comparable improvement in the number of rehabilitations.

In the material that follows we discuss service and result plans separately, but we recognize that combination plans are feasible. In discussing the advantages and disadvantages of each of these plans we make certain assumptions.

First, we assume that there is some annual limit or cap on expenditures for the BRP. Such a limit may be statutory, based upon a percentage of the benefit amounts, or it may be based, as the GAO has advocated, on a year-to-year assessment of the program's functioning. Later we can relax this assumption and suggest possible ways to determine the aggregate amount.

Second, we assume that beneficiaries who receive services from the state agencies are eligible to receive them, that is, they meet the four eligibility criteria. Our second assumption is necessary because the plans we will suggest, at least initially, are concerned with the allotment of funds to the states rather than the actual payment to the states. The distinction is an important one. Concern with allotment plans rather than plans of reimbursement for actual expenditure leads to our third assumption. This assumption is that allotments to a state agency, whether made on the basis of services rendered or on the basis of some measure of results, are used by those states as reimbursement for services rendered (and in light of our second assumption, services rendered to eligible clients).

There is a cash flow problem although we do not believe it to be a crucial one. A cash flow problem is common to all plans, including the one used currently. Funds are advanced to an agency subject to the presenting of vouchers for services rendered, and compensation is made for overhead and administrative costs based upon some documentation of these costs.

In our consideration of alternative financing plans, we will concentrate on the more conventional notion of allotments on the basis of various measures. Such allotments are maximum sums that can be spent by the states.

It is not possible to devise a plan that has a reasonable chance of meeting the equity, efficiency, and administrative convenience tests and that at the same time eliminates the need for all policing of the program. The various program administrative reviews (PARs) would not be displaced by any of these financing plans. The basic purposes of a financing plan are to ensure that the intentions of the legislature are carried out insofar as savings to the trust fund are concerned, to ensure that funds are properly conserved, and to create incentives for agencies to provide services to eligible clients. No plan can guarantee that only eligible clients will be served or that the program will continue to function well without administrative checks and balances.

Allotments Based Upon the Number of Rehabilitations

The Plan. One of the simpler alternative plans is to allot funds on the basis of the number of rehabilitations in each state. Eligible clients who successfully complete their individualized rehabilitation plans are closed in status 26, rehabilitated. The test for closure as a rehabilitant is placement in a job for a minimum of 60 days, and for DI trust fund financed cases, that job must be in competitive employment.

What changes would be made in the distribution of the BRP funds if the allotments were based on rehabilitations rather than on the DI beneficiary population? Table 1-7 shows the changes if the 1975 total allotments were distributed in accordance with the 1973 rehabilitations. The 2-year gap is chosen on the grounds that, realistically, the next year's allotments must be based on last year's records.

We recognize that one of the purposes of changing the financing plan is to affect the behavior of the agencies and to modify the incentive system under which they operate. In calculating the redistribution of funds, however, we must make use of the record of rehabilitations that were achieved under the present system.

We note that changes are considerable in individual states. About as many states would gain funds as would lose funds, and since we are redistributing a fixed sum, the amounts gained and lost are equal except for some rounding problems. In terms of absolute dollar changes, the big gainers are Minnesota, Ohio, and Texas. In terms of relative or percentage gains, Colorado, Minnesota, and North Dakota gain over 100 percent of their 1975 allotments. The losses are distributed more widely, with Michigan, Puerto Rico, and Tennessee each losing more than one-half million dollars. In relative terms, Arizona, D.C., Hawaii, Indiana, Kentucky, and Maine would lose 50 percent or more of their 1975 funds.

Obviously, if it were desirable to move to a system of

allotments according to rehabilitations, government could ease the transition by some guarantee that funding would not change more than a specified percentage in any one year.

While the adoption of a financing plan based on rehabilitations might lead to great changes in the funds available to particular states, it would not substantially alter the relative ranking of the states. Under the actual 1975 allotments, based on the number of beneficiaries in each state, California, New York, Pennsylvania, and Texas lead the list. If the funds were allocated to reflect the number of rehabilitations, California and New York would still rank in the top three states, although they would be joined by Ohio, which would assume the number one position.[21]

The coefficient of rank correlation as we change allotments in any of the plans presented ranges from the high 0.80s to the high 0.90s. This indicates that the population factor is powerful enough to dominate all other factors. The large states have more DI beneficiaries, more rehabilitations, and more terminations simply because they have greater populations.

The proposed plan does not pay a flat sum per rehabilitation, nor does it pay for the services afforded those people who have been rehabilitated. Instead it allots funds based on the number of rehabilitants. The number of rehabilitants is a comparative measure of the functioning of the individual agencies and is used to allocate funds. Those funds, once allotted, could be expended on eligible clients in accordance with the usual expenditure rules and regulations.

The Advantages. A financing plan based on rehabilitations would be consonant with the traditional goals of the vocational rehabilitation program. Counselors regard working toward the closure of their clients in a rehabilitated status as their principal task. They view rehabilitation as success, and closure in a nonrehabilitated status as failure, and they believe that the provision of services, counseling, guidance, and eventual placement contributes to the goal of the client's rehabilitation. Selection of clients, the devising of a plan for services, and the

Table 1-7 Reallocation of Allotments According to Rehabilitations

State or Territory	No. of Rehabs. FY 1973	Hypothetical Allotments According to Rehabs.*	Actual FY 1975 Initial State Allotments	Columns 3–4†
Alabama	134	$ 993,867	$ 1,871,534	−$877,667
Arizona	43	318,922	719,820	−400,898
Arkansas	126	934,537	1,259,686	−325,149
California	894	6,630,761	9,039,957	−2,409,196
Colorado	180	1,335,050	611,848	+723,202
Connecticut	93	689,770	935,767	−245,997
Delaware	28	207,673	179,956	+27,717
District of Columbia	14	103,837	251,937	−148,100
Florida	301	2,232,501	3,311,174	−1,078,673
Georgia	222	1,646,560	2,339,416	−692,856
Hawaii	12	88,996	179,956	−90,960
Idaho	63	467,264	329,597	+137,667
Illinois	822	6,096,738	3,419,147	+2,677,591
Indiana	98	726,856	1,799,551	−1,072,695
Iowa	179	1,327,630	899,776	+427,854
Kansas	103	763,941	647,838	+116,103
Kentucky	86	637,852	1,691,578	−1,053,726
Louisiana	142	1,053,206	1,763,560	−710,354
Maine	29	215,085	431,892	−216,807
Maryland	129	956,782	1,115,721	−158,939
Massachusetts	150	1,112,537	1,835,543	−723,006
Michigan	398	2,951,945	3,455,139	−503,194
Minnesota	422	3,129,953	1,043,740	+2,086,213
Mississippi	186	1,379,548	1,295,677	+83,871
Missouri	327	2,425,342	1,979,506	+445,936
Montana	52	385,681	251,937	+133,744
Nebraska	33	244,759	431,892	−187,133
Nevada	31	229,918	224,024	+5,894

BENEFICIARY REHABILITATION PROGRAM 37

(Table 1-7 continued)

New Hampshire	9	66,751	215,946	−149,195
New Jersey ‡				
New Mexico	89	660,105	412,184	+247,921
New York	853	6,326,664	6,730,321	−403,657
North Carolina	344	2,551,431	2,519,372	+32,059
North Dakota	70	519,183	221,855	+297,328
Ohio	932	6,912,605	3,851,040	+3,061,565
Oklahoma	149	1,105,124	1,223,695	−118,571
Oregon	126	934,537	935,767	−1,230
Pennsylvania	627	4,650,431	4,858,788	−208,357
Puerto Rico	126	934,537	1,583,605	−649,068
Rhode Island	27	200,253	359,910	−159,657
South Carolina	286	2,121,245	1,403,650	+717,595
South Dakota	32	237,338	215,946	+21,392
Tennessee	212	1,572,389	2,087,479	−515,090
Texas	695	5,154,781	3,887,031	+1,267,750
Utah	39	289,257	251,937	+37,320
Vermont	20	148,335	148,960	−625
Virginia	225	1,668,813	1,907,524	−238,711
Washington ‡				
West Virginia	201	1,490,805	1,367,659	+123,146
Wisconsin	300	2,225,081	1,511,623	+713,458
Wyoming	27	200,253	150,000	+50,253
Virgin Islands	1	7,412	25,000	−17,588
Alaska	13	96,416	150,000	−53,584
Guam	0	0	25,000	−25,000
Totals †	10,700	79,361,257	79,361,461	−204

*Hypothetical allotment for state$_i$ = $\frac{\text{\# of rehabilitations in state}_i}{\text{total \# of rehabilitations}}$ × 1975 total initial allotment.

† Differences in column totals due to rounding.

‡ States of New Jersey and Washington are excluded from all calculations due to omission of general agency rehabilitation data from R300 Tape.

Source: 1973 SRS-RSA R300 Tape and State Vocational Rehabilitation Agency Program Data, 1975.

offering and monitoring of these services are all directed towards this traditional goal.

Disadvantages. A time lag is inevitable in any scheme based upon results. One year's allotment will necessarily be based on the rehabilitations achieved one or two years prior to the year in question. In turn, these rehabilitations are frequently the outcome of services furnished in prior years. Still, the time lag under this scheme would not be as great as under the other plans that are based upon outcome measures.

A financing plan based on rehabilitations might also pose operational problems for the agencies. If the number of rehabilitations fluctuated greatly, rising sharply in one fiscal year and slackening off during the next year, funding would be correspondingly erratic. We ought to note, however, that the number of DI beneficiaries in a state may also fluctuate, and that it would be possible to devise a plan that limits these year-to-year fluctuations.

From the point of view of the agency, the greatest disadvantage of this scheme is that it is not an allotment based directly upon services rendered or upon the effort expended by agency personnel in carrying out their daily tasks.

Evaluation. Because all rehabilitants do not terminate, a system of payments on the basis of rehabilitations may not be optimally efficient. Net savings to the trust fund can differ across rehabilitations. On the other hand, rehabilitations do bear a closer relationship to terminations and savings to the trust fund than do services provided or allotments on the basis of some population measure.

The plan is probably neutral with regard to equity considerations. Whatever restrictions are placed on selecting clients or providing services because the eventual goal is rehabilitation are shared by the general program as well. It is likely that one could order any type of priority selection and still not abandon the plan of allotments based upon rehabilitations.

The plan is also administratively feasible. Although there is the necessary one- or two-year time lag, data as to the number of rehabilitations are readily available.

A system of allotments based on the number of rehabilitations would require some form of program review to assure that only eligible clients were classified as rehabilitants under the plan and that these rehabilitants were placed in competitive employment. It would have the advantage of moving the system towards a more efficient point by focusing on the result or outcome and not necessarily on the services.

Payments on the Basis of Terminations

The Plan. Another plan would allot funds in accordance with the number of rehabilitants who have terminated from the disability beneficiary rolls. Termination occurs when a beneficiary has earnings from employment that exceed the substantial gainful activity (SGA) level or if his or her medical condition improves. The fact of medical recovery can be certified by administrative decision of the SSA; in such cases, the SSA orders benefits to be terminated. Benefits may also be terminated if the individual refuses the appropriate tendering of vocational rehabilitation services, although such terminations have been rare.

In Table 1-8, we list terminations through 1976 of all cases which the agencies closed rehabilitated in fiscal 1973, as determined by a search of the social security records. Table 1-8 shows the 1975 actual allotments and the allotments that would have been made had they been based on these terminations. Such an allotment plan would work in much the same way as the plan based on rehabilitations. Once the number of terminations is known, the federal government could allocate monies among the states in accordance with the proportionate number of terminations recorded for each state of the total number of terminations. The money would be allotted to the states to be used for reimbursement of services offered to DI beneficiaries eligible for trust fund financing during the current fiscal year.

Advantages. Although the net savings that accrue to the trust

Table 1-8 Reallocation of Allotments According to Termination of 1973 BRP Rehabilitations

1 State or Territory	2 No. of Terminations of 1973 BRP Rehabs*	3 Hypothetical Allotments According to Terminations of 1973 BRP Rehabs†	4 Actual FY 1975 Initial State Allotments	5 Columns 3–4
Alabama	23	$ 782,054	$ 1,871,534	−$1,089,480
Arizona	15	510,035	719,820	−209,785
Arkansas	8	272,019	1,259,686	−987,667
California	329	11,186,770	9,039,957	+2,146,813
Colorado	41	1,394,096	611,848	+782,248
Connecticut	28	952,066	935,767	+16,299
Delaware	10	340,023	179,956	+160,067
District of Columbia	2	68,005	251,937	−183,932
Florida	84	2,856,197	3,311,174	−454,977
Georgia	75	2,550,176	2,339,416	+210,760
Hawaii	3	102,007	179,956	−77,949
Idaho	19	646,044	329,597	+316,447
Illinois	124	4,216,290	3,419,147	+797,143
Indiana	25	850,059	1,799,551	−949,492
Iowa	47	1,598,110	899,776	+698,334
Kansas	28	952,066	647,838	+304,228
Kentucky	22	748,051	1,691,578	−943,527
Louisiana	28	952,066	1,763,560	−811,494
Maine	9	306,021	431,892	−125,871
Maryland	19	646,044	1,115,721	−469,677
Massachusetts	36	1,224,084	1,835,543	−611,459
Michigan	136	4,624,318	3,455,139	+1,169,179
Minnesota	53	1,802,124	1,043,740	+758,384
Mississippi	31	1,054,073	1,295,677	−241,604
Missouri	68	2,312,159	1,979,506	+332,653
Montana	10	340,023	251,937	+88,086
Nebraska	11	374,026	431,892	−57,866
Nevada	6	204,014	224,024	−26,010

(Table 1-8 continued)

New Hampshire	3	102,007	215,946	−113,939
New Jersey ‡	6	—	—	—
New Mexico	17	578,040	412,184	+165,856
New York	158	5,372,370	6,730,321	−1,357,951
North Carolina	73	2,482,171	2,519,372	−37,201
North Dakota	15	510,035	221,855	+288,180
Ohio	142	4,828,332	3,851,040	+977,292
Oklahoma	19	646,044	1,223,695	−577,651
Oregon	33	1,122,077	935,767	+186,310
Pennsylvania	131	4,454,307	4,858,788	−404,481
Puerto Rico	3	102,007	1,583,605	−1,481,598
Rhode Island	5	170,012	359,910	−189,898
South Carolina	69	2,346,161	1,403,650	+942,511
South Dakota	5	170,012	215,946	−45,934
Tennessee	44	1,496,103	2,087,479	−591,376
Texas	124	4,216,290	3,887,031	+329,259
Utah	18	612,042	251,937	+360,105
Vermont	4	136,009	148,960	−12,951
Virginia	47	1,598,110	1,907,524	−309,414
Washington ‡	1	—	—	—
West Virginia	35	1,190,082	1,367,659	−177,577
Wisconsin	88	2,992,206	1,511,623	+1,480,583
Wyoming	3	102,007	150,000	−47,993
Virgin Islands	1	34,002	25,000	+9,002
Alaska	0	0	150,000	−150,000
Guam	0	0	25,000	−25,000
Totals §	2,327	79,361,524	79,361,461	+63

*Terminations include only those 1973 BRP rehabilitations with both an MBR and an R-300 record who left the DI beneficiary rolls because of recovery for any duration during the period January 1973 to January 1977.

†Hypothetical allotment for state$_i$ = $\frac{\text{\# of terminations of 1973 BRP rehabilitations for state}_i}{\text{total \# of terminations of 1973 BRP rehabilitations}}$ × 1975 total initial allotment.

‡States of New Jersey and Washington are excluded from all calculations as a result of omission of general agency rehabilitation data from R-300 tape.

§ Differences in column totals due to rounding.

Source: 1973 SRS-RSA R-300 Tape, SSA Master Beneficiary Records, and State Vocational Rehabilitation Agency Program Data, 1975.

fund as a result of terminations cannot be calculated without cost information and information on relapses, a financing plan based on terminations has the clear advantage of linking the allotment of funds to the goal of net savings. If the intent of Congress in providing BRP funds was in fact to remove people from the beneficiary rolls, then such a plan clearly advances this objective.

Termination is a certain indication that a person has left the DI rolls. As a measure of output, it is definitive. Consequently, this concept is preferable to rehabilitation, which is a judgmental measure based upon wage data and upon a subjective evaluation of a client's status.

Disadvantages. To link financing to terminations is to compensate agencies for a result that they may be unable to control. It can be argued that the rehabilitation agency's job is to rehabilitate clients, and that whether or not the beneficiary terminates may be due to a host of factors which the agency's work cannot affect.

Evaluation. Since terminations, more so than rehabilitations, are closely related to savings to the trust fund, a scheme based on terminations rates higher on efficiency grounds than one based upon rehabilitations.

Grave equity considerations are involved in basing allotments on terminations. Such a system may create an incentive to serve first those who are less severely disabled or those who show the greatest probability of termination. In addition, the agency that showed a greater ability to terminate clients would receive a greater amount of funds. The departure from the present system of distribution based upon population may violate some notions of equity, even as it serves the ends of efficiency.

The administrative feasibility of the plan raises other questions. It would be easy for government to ascertain the number of terminations in any given fiscal year and to use this information as a guide in allocating funds. However, we have stressed that one important purpose of a financing plan is to provide incentives to the individuals currently working in the program; in other words, to reward agencies that have a successful rehabilitation record and to penalize those that have not done well. Under a plan that depends on termination data, it would be very difficult to administer rewards and penalties promptly enough to ensure that they had the intended incentive (or disincentive) effect. Terminations in any one fiscal year are based upon rehabilitations of the preceding year or years, and these rehabilitations, in turn, may be based upon services rendered several years earlier. Over such an extended period of time, agency personnel may change, and new organizational structures may arise within an agency. Agency personnel of 1978 might find themselves being rewarded or penalized for the activities of their predecessors in, for example, 1973. This time lag problem is probably the greatest single weakness of the allotment plan based on terminations.

Table 1-8 shows the reallotment according to the termination measure. Again we note that the relative ranking of states does not change drastically. The coefficient of rank correlation between ranking by terminations and by the 1975 allotments is 0.882. If we consider the ranking according to terminations and the ranking according to rehabilitations, the coefficient increases to 0.945. In both bases, the factor influencing the ranking is relative population.

Changes in individual states are considerable, however. In dollar terms the greatest gainer is California, followed by Michigan, Wisconsin, and Ohio. New York and two smaller jurisdictions, Alabama and Puerto Rico, are the large losers. We can gain only a limited amount of information from these reallotments because they are based on past records made at a time when allotments were on a population basis. The idea behind any alternative plan is to influence agencies to adopt different patterns of behavior. Had the plan been in effect, it may have had the result of changing behavior, and consequently, the reallotments might have been different.

Payments Based Upon Savings to the Trust Fund

The Plan. The third and final plan we propose is one in which funds would be allotted to the states according to estimates of actual savings. Such a system would be directly on target, with each state receiving a proportionate amount of the sum allocated according to its proportionate share of savings.

Using information on individual characteristics and DI benefits and the same assumptions given above, we can estimate the savings to the fund occasioned by each beneficiary's termination. Following the procedure we adopted with rehabilitations and terminations, we can use each state's proportionate share of the savings to redistribute the 1975 allotments (Table 1-9), together with actual 1975 state allotments and the differences. As with our other measures, the relative rankings are changed, but not drastically. The changes in individual states are considerable. California would now lead the states by a wide margin. The savings due to its 273 terminations would entitle it to $150 per $1,000 of the total allotment. New York is the second state in rank according to the savings criterion—the same position it held under the 1975 formula—but it would receive less than one-half of California's share, or $64 per $1,000 of allotment. Pennsylvania, the third ranking state under the current plan, drops one notch and Ohio assumes the number three position.

Instead of allotting to states a predetermined fixed sum based upon a percentage of last year's benefits, it would be possible with the savings plan to fix the total sum according to the present value of the savings. The cap on aggregate expenditures for the coming year could be determined by the savings of the previous year. Essentially, all the plans considered above entailed redistributing a fixed sum. Such redistribution is a type of zero-sum game; because some states gain, others must lose. Allotting according to rehabilitations, terminations, or proportionate savings does not give any hint as to how much might be spent on the program as a whole. The savings calculation, on the other hand, yields a dollar amount that could be used to fix the aggregate amount to be distributed.

Admittedly the program's financing might be drastically reduced. If the FY 1973 savings had been used in fiscal 1975, the program would have distributed $49 million to the states instead of $79 million. But here we offer the same caution as in our evaluations of the other plans. Had such a plan been in effect it might have altered the behavior of the actors in the program. In other words, if it had been made clear that the prime objective was to increase aggregate savings, more funds might have been saved. The purpose of a new plan would be to change the rules and to motivate the participants in new directions. Changes might have to be made gradually, however, lest programs that have evolved over the years are discarded without the participants having being given an opportunity to play by the new rules.

Advantages. The prime advantage of such a plan is that it estimates the actual savings to the trust fund. If one of the purposes of the BRP is to reduce overall trust fund expenditures by restoring people to gainful employment, then saving is an ideal measure of the extent to which the program has succeeded. It takes into account the fact that the savings to the fund caused by each rehabilitation and eventual termination may differ by quite a bit.

Disadvantages. All of the disadvantages of plans based on rehabilitations and terminations recur in the plan based on savings, but in an even more exaggerated form. Savings to the fund are more removed in time than either rehabilitations or terminations from the actual provision of services. Furthermore, the rehabilitation agency has even less control of savings than they do of terminations. As we suggested earlier, whether or not a person terminates is certainly not independent of the quality of the rehabilitation, but services alone do not account for the outcome in any particular case. Whether a person's termination is going to result in little or great savings depends on the level of benefits he or she had been receiving, the continuing availability of alternative earning opportunities, the person's physical condition over time, and many other factors outside the influence of rehabilitation agencies. Although agencies have the right to follow a person after he or she has reached a rehabilitated status, it goes beyond their traditional concern to influence his termination decision or to inquire into his legal position with regard to a

Table 1-9 Reallocation of Allotments According to Savings to DI Trust Fund

State or Territory	No. of Single Terminations of 1973 BRP Rehabs.*	Present Value of Savings to DI Trust Fund From Single Terminations of 1973 BRP Rehabs.†	Hypothetical Allotments According to Present Value of Savings‡	Actual FY 1975 Initial State Allotments	Columns 4–5
Alabama	20	$ 596,559	$ 971,622	$ 1,871,534	−$ 899,912
Alaska	0	0	0	150,000	−150,000
Arizona	14	373,675	608,607	719,820	−111,213
Arkansas	6	75,255	122,566	1,259,686	−1,137,120
California	273	7,335,575	11,947,535	9,039,957	+2,907,578
Colorado	32	635,864	1,035,643	611,848	+422,795
Connecticut	23	636,254	1,036,270	935,767	+100,503
Delaware	7	192,679	313,811	179,956	+133,855
District of Columbia	1	49,554	80,703	251,937	−171,234
Florida	64	1,591,198	2,591,596	3,311,174	−719,578
Georgia	63	1,583,971	2,579,827	2,339,416	+240,411
Hawaii	2	89,749	146,168	179,956	−33,788
Idaho	18	438,361	713,960	329,597	+384,363
Illinois	98	2,766,925	4,506,517	3,419,147	+1,087,370
Indiana	19	425,666	693,286	1,799,551	−1,106,265
Iowa	39	1,069,419	1,741,770	899,776	+841,994
Kansas	25	610,308	994,010	647,838	+346,172
Kentucky	19	349,205	568,752	1,691,578	−1,122,826
Louisiana	21	557,477	907,967	1,763,560	−855,593
Maine	8	206,161	335,770	431,892	−96,122
Maryland	16	304,707	496,279	1,115,721	−619,442
Massachusetts	31	881,258	1,435,308	1,835,543	−400,235
Michigan	118	4,131,130	6,728,415	3,455,139	+3,273,276
Minnesota	44	1,266,337	2,062,493	1,043,740	+1,018,753
Mississippi	23	469,343	764,418	1,295,677	−531,259
Missouri	53	1,135,294	1,847,432	1,979,506	−132,074
Montana	10	157,348	256,274	251,937	+4,337
Nebraska	10	281,592	458,630	431,892	+26,738
Nevada	5	175,560	285,931	224,024	+61,907
New Hampshire	2	33,704	54,886	215,946	−161,060

(Table 1-9 continued)

New Jersey§	—	—	—	—	—
New Mexico	14	448,887	731,102	412,184	+319,118
New York	126	3,099,919	5,048,873	6,730,321	−1,681,448
North Carolina	55	1,245,774	2,029,003	2,519,372	−492,369
North Dakota	11	180,464	293,923	221,855	+72,068
Ohio	106	2,707,636	4,409,958	3,851,040	+558,918
Oklahoma	16	492,538	802,202	1,223,695	−421,493
Oregon	25	701,022	1,141,757	935,767	+205,990
Pennsylvania	100	2,639,152	4,298,415	4,858,788	−560,373
Puerto Rico	2	60,066	97,829	1,583,605	−1,485,776
Rhode Island	5	177,316	288,796	359,910	−71,114
South Carolina	58	341,606	2,185,083	1,403,650	+781,433
South Dakota	5	106,617	173,643	215,946	−42,303
Tennessee	34	779,758	1,269,998	2,087,479	−817,481
Texas	105	2,493,814	4,061,704	3,887,031	+174,673
Utah	17	347,915	566,649	251,937	+314,712
Vermont	4	85,514	139,271	148,960	−9,689
Virginia	40	971,545	1,582,364	1,907,524	−325,160
Washington§	—	—	—	—	—
West Virginia	33	698,015	1,136,861	1,367,659	230,798
Wisconsin	73	1,662,247	2,707,321	1,511,623	+1,195,698
Wyoming	2	68,430	111,447	150,000	−38,553
Virgin Islands	0	0	0	25,000	−25,000
Guam	0	0	0	25,000	−25,000
Totals//	1,892	48,726,515	79,361,645	79,361,461	+184

*Single terminations include only those 1973 BRP rehabilitations with both an MBR and 1973 R300 record who terminated due to recovery following rehabilitation and had not returned to the DI benefit rolls as of January 1977.

†Present value of savings in current dollars is computed as of the year of termination using the primary insurance amount as a proxy for the primary beneficiary's monthly benefit amount and the family maximum as a proxy for the actual monthly family benefit amount. Recidivists and multiple terminations are not included in the estimates of savings. For those BRP rehabilitants who terminated in FY 1977, savings were estimated using June 1976 as the termination date.

‡Hypothetical allotment for state$_i$ = $\frac{\text{present value of savings for state}_i}{\text{total present value of savings}}$ × 1975 total initial allotment.

§States of New Jersey and Washington are excluded from all calculations due to omission of general agency rehabilitation data from R300 Tape.

//Differences in column totals due to rounding.

Source: 1973 SRS-RSA R300 Tape, State Vocational Rehabilitation Agency Program Data, 1975 and SSA Master Beneficiary Records.

particular benefit program. It is also beyond their power to control the economic and demographic factors that influence savings.

Evaluation. The plan scores high from an efficiency point of view. Whether the amount of savings recorded is merely a standard to allocate funds to the states on a proportional basis, or whether allotments are made equivalent to actual savings, we are dealing with a measure that is intimately related to the efficiency objective of savings to the fund.

Such a plan probably ranks low on most equity scales. If the agencies were influenced by savings criteria exclusively, they would concentrate on selecting as clients those people who could be expected to show the greatest savings. Agency preferences would be directed toward the younger person, the person with the greatest number of dependents, and the person who was most likely to terminate on a permanent basis. Such considerations might well conflict with equity standards; the older severely handicapped person could be pushed far back in the queue.

The plan would have some administrative difficulties. Reasonable people might differ about the assumptions used in deciding upon discount rates, rates of inflation, mortality rates, probabilities of recidivism, and any of the other variables. To substitute actual experience for estimates would make the scheme thoroughly unworkable, because some program planners would have to wait many years before actual results could be obtained.

If a consensus is reached or the appropriate estimate of these variables, we are still faced with the fact that a plan based on savings to the trust fund would entail allotting funds to agencies on the basis of their performance in rehabilitating clients years earlier. As a result, any incentive effects from using this plan would be greatly diminished. It may be possible to devise proxies for the savings figures, but a procedure that would replace the actual calculation of the aggregate savings would be difficult to formulate.

A Review of the Plans

The current plan, based upon the relative number of DI beneficiaries in a state, ranks lowest in efficiency terms. It is a population-based measure that is not even remotely connected to any efficiency measure. The fact that the BRP functions as well as it does is a tribute to the vocational rehabilitation agencies and not to the allotment plan. The current plan does have, however, the great advantage of giving each DI beneficiary in a state an equal share of the potential rehabilitation funds.

The plan that ranks third in efficiency is the one in which allotments are geared to the number of rehabilitants. Rehabilitation is a measure of results achieved, and it is the necessary prerequisite for terminations. Consequently, we rank terminations second and savings to the trust fund first in efficiency among the plans considered.

Savings to the fund is the most desirable measure of results, but a plan based upon savings has the possible defect of funding agencies for services rendered at a much earlier point in time. In order to correct this defect, we must devise a proxy for savings to the fund that would be available in reasonable time. We have calculated the estimated present value of savings in Table 1-9 in the interest of determining whether the present system of allotments by DI beneficiary populations is a reasonably good predictor of savings. Inspection of Table 1-9 shows considerable changes in amounts allotted to individual states, but no great difference in relative rankings.

The simple coefficient of correlation between the savings by states and allotments by states is high, 0.91, but of course population factors would account for the close relationship. It is possible to eliminate the influence of population by deflating the dollar amounts by the actual population of the states and calculating the allotments per 1,000 population and the savings per 1,000 population in each state. When we do so, the coefficient of correlation drops drastically and it is not significantly different from zero. The principal explanation for the drop is that the allotment measure is already based upon population. Without further tests, we can conclude that there simply is no relationship between the current method of allotments and savings to the fund. Such a conclusion reinforces our prior estimate of the low ranking of the present system on an efficiency scale.

Our next candidate for a proxy measure is rehabilitations. The rehabilitation count is a traditional measure and is available in reasonable time. Rehabilitations by states and savings by states are closely related (coefficient of correlation is 0.87) when no account is taken of population differences. When we divide by population, however, the coefficient drops but only to 0.65, which shows a fairly strong relationship between rehabilitation and savings.

As an alternative, we might consider a "higher quality" rehabilitation, defining quality in terms of wage at closure. There exists a direct (and not surprising) relationship between wage at closure and termination.

The simplest measure to consider is rehabilitation at a wage greater than the SGA level, which was $140 a month in 1973. Available data show that about 24 percent of all rehabilitants terminate. But if we confine our consideration to rehabilitations at a wage greater than SGA, we find that 38 percent terminate. In other words, over 90 percent of all terminations were persons who were rehabilitated at a wage at SGA levels or greater.

The number of SGA rehabilitations is a significantly better predictor of savings than all rehabilitations. The simple coefficient of correlation between rehabilitation and savings, both deflated by population, was 0.65; substituting the SGA measure for rehabilitations improves the coefficient to 0.77.

Implementing a Financing Plan

We are now in the position to put forth the basic components of a new financing method for the BRP. Although our emphasis is on efficiency, we recognize that an ideal plan will take equity considerations into account and will be practical from an administrative viewpoint. In designing our plan, we have held ourselves to two conditions: that as much weight as possible be given to the best available proxy for savings, and that aggregate expenditures should eventually be limited by aggregate savings.

Timing. Drastic changes in the way the present system is financed might create confusion and jeopardize the effective functioning of the program. One way to avoid problems would be to freeze the current level of funding as the new plan is being put into effect, allowing only for changes as a result of price level movements. Other changes should go into effect gradually, over as long a period as the administration of the system will permit.

Allotment Criteria. The plan combines essentially two measures, one that ranks reasonably high on efficiency grounds and a second that is compatible with a wide variety of equity notions.

With regard to the second, we reject measures based on case services, administration costs, or categories of clients. Although such criteria might measure agency effort, they could not assess the results of rehabilitation efforts. Because we recognize, however, that a wide variety of clients should be served, we desire a measure sensitive to equity considerations. We choose the traditional DI population measure, although we would weigh it heavily only during the period when the new financing plan is introduced and the system is in transition.

As for the efficiency measure, we would choose rehabilitations at a wage equal to or greater than the SGA limit. We would not reward rehabilitations at wages too low to terminate.

Phasing in the Plan. In order to demonstrate how the plan might work, we choose a phasing in period of 7 years. During the first year, we would allocate three-quarters of the funds by the method that is currently in use. The remaining quarter of the funds would be allocated according to the proportionate number of SGA rehabilitations in the latest year available.

During the second year, we propose that funding be on a 50-50 basis, weighting DI population and SGA rehabilitations equally. During the third year, the proportions would be 25 percent for the DI population and 75 percent for SGA rehabilitations; that division would continue in the following years.

During the first, second, and third years the annual aggregate amount would be constant save for price level adjustments.

Annual Expenditure Limits. We propose that, beginning in the fourth year, the savings in the aggregate be used to set the amounts to be appropriated for the program. We believe that the new method of setting the cap on the program should be instituted gradually.

During that year, the aggregate amount to be allotted would be determined by taking a major proportion, for example, three-quarters, of the prior year's allotment, after adjusting for price changes. To that sum would be added some proportion, for example, one-quarter, of the prior year's aggregate savings. The total amount derived from taking a proportion of last year's allotment and a proportion of savings would then be allocated to the states according to the 75 percent SGA and 25 percent DI formula used in the third year. Note that the total amount in the fourth year could be greater or less than in the third year, depending on proportions chosen and the size of the savings amount.

In the fifth year, the same procedure would be repeated, but now a smaller proportion, e.g., 50 percent, of the base year (that is, the third year's amount) would be used with a larger proportion, e.g., 50 percent, of last year's (fourth year) savings, suitably adjusted for price changes. In the sixth year, an even smaller proportion, e.g., 25 percent, of the base year's allotment, as adjusted, is used and possibly 75 percent of the fifth year's savings. In the seventh year, 100 percent of the prior year's savings is used as a cap on expenditures. Such a cap might be retained until some future date when individual measures of efficiency might make any ceiling unnecessary. Such a gradual change would give the system a chance to adjust to the new measures of success. The rudiments of an ideal plan are summarized in Table 1-10.

Reimbursing Expenditures. As with any other financing plan, this scheme can work only if other elements of the BRP are working properly. If the special selection criteria are well

Table 1-10
Rudiments of an Ideal Financing Plan

Year*	Determination of Cap on Total Allotment	Determination of a State's Initial Allotment
1		1. A share of *75%* of the total allotment based upon a state's proportionate share of *DI beneficiaries*. 2. A share of *25%* of the total allotment based upon a state's proportionate share of *SGA rehabilitations*.
2	Frozen at current level with adjustments for price changes.	1. A share of *50%* of the total allotment based upon a state's proportionate share of *DI beneficiaries*. 2. A share of *50%* of the total allotment based upon a state's proportionate share of *SGA rehabilitations*.
3		
4	75% of third year's total allotment plus 25% of aggregate savings in previous year.	
5	50% of third year's total allotment plus 50% of aggregate savings in previous year.	1. A share of *25%* of the total allotment based upon a state's proportionate share of *DI beneficiaries*. 2. A share of *75%* of the total allotment based upon a state's proportionate share of *SGA rehabilitations*.
6	25% of third year's total allotment plus 75% of aggregate savings in previous year.	
7	100% of aggregate savings in previous year.	

* The seven-year periods are used for illustrative purposes only.

monitored, then the sums allotted to the states could be used as they are at present, for reimbursement of expenditures on current clients. If audits of cases show a poor selection of cases, however, then we must consider alternative plans under which states are compensated at a flat amount for each SGA rehabilitation or termination, or are compensated dollar for dollar of proven savings.

Conclusion

In this section, we have proposed a method for financing the BRP that virtually guarantees that the program will be permanently cost-beneficial. The financing scheme is, in effect, self-correcting; if the savings to the trust fund from terminations fall below the cost of the program, the size of the program would be automatically reduced until the ratio of savings to costs becomes equal to or greater than one. Obviously, such a reduction in the size of the BRP is only a fail-safe device. Our intention is that the BRP should grow as it produces greater savings to the trust fund and serves more and more beneficiaries.

Thus, regardless of the financing method used the question remains of how the current operation of the BRP can be altered to improve its performance. With respect to benefits and costs, the solution is twofold: first, a more efficient application of the special selection criteria for identifying BRP clients is needed; and second, disincentives to terminate, which may exist in the structure of the program, must be reduced. The two remedies are related, because by eliminating disincentives, the likelihood that any given beneficiary will terminate will be enhanced. Consequently, the population that meets the special selection criteria will be larger. These issues are taken up in the following section.

IMPROVING PROGRAM PERFORMANCE: CLIENT SELECTION AND INCENTIVES

The success of the BRP depends not only on the method of allocating funds to the states but also on the effectiveness of counselors in helping people leave the DI rolls. Counselor effectiveness, in turn, is limited by such independent factors as the characteristics of the clients and the structure of the DI program. Changes in DI rules and regulations along with changes in the method and criteria of client selection may improve counselor and program performance.

As with so many other disability programs, the DI program presents a classical dilemma. Up to the point where an applicant gains admission to the program, all of his incentives are to maximize the extent of his physical or mental disabilities in order to qualify for benefits. Yet the whole purpose of the BRP is to emphasize the client's residual capabilities so that he can leave the rolls and return to the labor force.

Counselors in the traditional rehabilitation program recognize these problems and have tended to prefer clients who may be easier to rehabilitate and who, once rehabilitated, may be left to pursue their own goals. The traditional goal of the vocational rehabilitation program is to close clients in the rehabilitated status. In the BRP, counselors must also be concerned with whether or not the rehabilitated person terminates from the DI rolls. Termination, however, is a function of variables over which the rehabilitation counselor may not have full control.

We contend, however, that the method of selecting clients for the BRP can be improved. The BRP can concentrate its limited resources on those persons whose rehabilitation would yield the greatest net savings to the trust fund. It can recognize the potential disincentive problems posed by the DI program, and formulate individual written rehabilitation plans with these problems in mind.

In this section we want to examine what has loosely been termed the *disincentive problem*. We want to determine whether there are factors in the BRP and the DI program which mitigate against termination. We have divided the analysis into two parts. In the first part, we look at the referral or the acceptance problem. Who should be admitted into the BRP? How should they be selected? The four selection criteria we outlined at the beginning of the chapter in essence describe a candidate who, after receiving services, will have a reasonable chance of being placed in a job earning an income that will lead to the termination of benefits. After a brief review of the criteria, we look at some of the characteristics of beneficiaries at the time of referral to the rehabilitation agency and the rates of eventual termination by characteristic. Second, we take a close look at the wage-to-benefit ratio, and the corresponding rate of termination. Finally, the characteristics are brought together in a probability of termination regression model. The model results provide some guidelines for improving the efficiency of the selection process. In the second part of our analysis, we examine possible disincentives that are built into the DI program.

Special Selection Criteria

Congress clearly expected the BRP to engage in a selection process and to subject the results of that process to continuous evaluation. The first special selection criterion "screens in" beneficiaries who are severely disabled but whose disability is not so rapidly progressive so as to outrun the effects of rehabilitation services or preclude restoration to productive activity. This criterion poses few problems. The program administrative review (PAR) cases indicate that it was met in over 95 percent of the cases.

The second special selection criterion requires that the disability be expected to remain at a level of severity that would result in continuing payment of disability benefits. In short, the beneficiary is not expected to recover spontaneously or without the services of vocational rehabilitation.

The GAO report found the application of this criterion to be a significant problem. Vocational rehabilitation services were taking credit for cases that would have terminated even without the services. A reasonable solution seems to be that vocational rehabilitation personnel ought not to be required to make decisions about the applicability of the criterion. The Disability

Determination Service Unit or the Rehabilitation Unit within the SSA could assume the responsibility of making the decisions.

Special selection criteria 3 and 4 are quite different from the first two. The expertise of the vocational rehabilitation counselor should clearly come into play in making these decisions. Special selection criterion 3 requires that there be a reasonable expectation that providing the vocational rehabilitation services will result in restoration of the individual to productive activity, and criterion 4 requires a type of individual benefit-cost analysis. The predictable period of productive work should be long enough so that the benefits will offset the cost of planned services.

The application of criteria 3 and 4 can be improved with data on how different client characteristics relate to success. Some understanding of these complex relationships can be garnered from a review of clients who were rehabilitated and subsequently left the rolls. There were 8,286 beneficiaries who were closed rehabilitated in FY 1973. Of this group, 2,938 individuals or approximately 35 percent of those rehabilitated in FY 1973 left the DI rolls at least once by January 1977.

Ideally, we would calculate the probability of termination based upon characteristics at the time of referral for all beneficiaries. If the counselor charged with applying criteria 3 and 4 had a reliable set of probabilities before him, applicable to the population he had to evaluate, then his job would be a relatively simple one of calculating expected net savings. A useful experiment could be devised that would collect the necessary information on the characteristics and outcomes of the relevant population, apply the methodology we use below to calculate the probability of termination, and select an experimental group for BRP services using an expected net savings criterion.

An important point should be made concerning the findings detailed in this chapter. The sample of DI beneficiaries we used to calculate the rates and probabilities of termination is one that includes only those that were referred, accepted, and rehabilitated under the BRP. Our results, then, are based upon a population that has already been through the selection process and not upon the population that is initially referred to vocational rehabilitation. For this reason, our results are only applicable as a means of improving the efficiency of the *current* selection process and are not meant as a substitute for the application of the special selection criteria.

Age

One of the factors that is associated with termination is the individual's age at the time of referral. The available data indicate that the likelihood of termination decreases the older the rehabilitant. Over 40 percent of the rehabilitants in the prime age group 25–34 terminate, and more than one-third of those in the 35–44 years age group also leave the rolls. By contrast, 14 percent of rehabilitants aged 55–64 terminate and none of those aged 65 years and over terminate. At age 65, DI recipients leave the rolls and transfer to the retirement program. The few rehabilitants aged 65 and over undoubtedly began the program at an earlier age.

Several reasons can explain the indicated relationship between age and termination. The older worker may have lower expectations concerning wage increases and promotions. The incidence and severity of disabling conditions accelerates with age, and employers may be reluctant to hire beneficiaries who are close to retirement age. Conversely, the younger workers' expectations may be high with respect to opportunities for advancement and higher salaries, and they face fewer barriers to employment.

The evidence suggests that the investment in rehabilitation may be more productive the younger the age of the worker. Because the younger worker has many years remaining to him as a member of the labor force, he has more incentive to leave the rolls and to reap returns on the investment in restoration or training. The BRP stands to gain as well by selecting younger clients: The younger the worker, the greater the savings in removing him from the benefit rolls.

Education

Another characteristic known to the counselor at the time of referral is the beneficiary's education. Approximately 28 percent of those rehabilitated in 1973 had no formal education beyond 8th grade. Of the 2,368 rehabilitants who fall into this group, 595 terminated. This amounts to a termination rate of approximately 25 percent, 10 percentage points below the average for the whole sample.

The termination rate improves to 34 percent for individuals with 1 to 3 years of high school and 41 percent for high school graduates. Education beyond high school does not significantly improve the chances of termination.

The positive influence of education on the rate of termination is to be expected. Education is traditionally used as a measure of the value of human capital: the greater the value of human capital the higher the wage the individual can command in the labor market.

Education also broadens the scope of an individual's knowledge and makes him more adaptable to change. The onset of disability may make it impossible for a person to return to his previous line of work and the better educated individual may make an easier adjustment to a new working situation.

Impairments and Pathology

There is no *a priori* reason to expect one type of impairment or illness to be associated with a higher or lower than average termination rate. Severity of impairment and the consequent functional limitations may be the important variables. We cannot determine, however, the severity of the impairment or the functional limitation from the available data sources. It is generally accepted that one must look at the interaction of the impairment and the consequent functional limitations with other factors such as age and education to determine whether a given impairment is disabling. We will attempt to control for these other factors later using regression techniques, but we cannot supply the missing information as to severity of impairments or functional limitation rates by substituting type of impairment or condition classification. Given these caveats we note that mentally retarded persons; persons with visual, hearing, and speech impairments; and persons with allergic, endocrine, metabolic, and nutritional diseases had lower than average rates of termination.

Race and Sex

The probability of termination is not significantly affected by the race of the rehabilitant. Predictably, however, sex is an important factor — probably because of the historically stronger attachment of the male to the labor force; 38 percent of males who were rehabilitated went on to terminate, as opposed to only 23.2 percent of all female rehabilitants.

Using sex as a selection factor is, however, questionable on two grounds. First, it may violate the antidiscrimination laws. Second, the data are for 1973 rehabilitants, and trends in the labor force since then show an increasing participation rate for women.

Marital Status

BRP rehabilitants who are married have only a slightly higher termination rate than the nonmarried rehabilitants. Married individuals have been shown in other studies to have higher participation rates. Married persons are also eligible for dependent benefits, however, and this may counteract incentives to terminate.

Characteristics at Time of Closure: Wage-Benefit Ratios

Information about basic demographic characteristics could be used to increase the efficiency of the selection process. Once clients are selected, the counselor provides services with the intent of increasing that individual's productive potential so that he or she can be placed in a job and closed successfully rehabilitated. As we have seen, however, rehabilitation does not guarantee termination and savings to the trust fund. An important variable is the quality of rehabilitation resulting from the services received. The measure of the quality of rehabilitation that we have chosen is the wage the individual earns at closure. Several cautions must be noted. Our information is based on the wage the client receives from a job held for the first sixty days. We cannot conclude from these data whether the rehabilitant was able to continue at his or her job beyond that period of time. Consequently, we expect that some relatively high wage workers closed at low wages may improve their labor market position and eventually terminate.

A necessary condition for termination is that monthly earnings equal or exceed the SGA level which was $140 a month or $32 a week in 1973. As shown in Table 1-11, a small percentage of rehabilitants who leave the rolls were closed at a wage less than the SGA level. These could be cases for which termination was the result of medical recovery. Or, as we suggested earlier, the closure wage of the individual could have increased, or he may have been able to locate a different job paying a wage greater than SGA.

It is apparent from the data in Table 1-11 that most individuals in this group are rehabilitated at wages above the SGA level. Some 23 percent of the rehabilitants were placed in jobs earning a weekly wage of $113 or better, which translates into monthly earnings of $500 or more. Why then do 40 percent of

Table 1-11
Wages at Closure and Rate of Termination

Weekly Wage at Closure	Category Total*	Nonterminations	Terminations†	Rate of Terminations
$ 0	2,104 (25.1)	2,006	98	4.7
1–16	486 (5.8)	466	20	4.1
17–32	713 (8.5)	636	77	10.8
33–48	467 (5.6)	350	117	25.1
49–64	574 (6.8)	373	201	35.0
65–80	861 (10.3)	428	433	50.3
81–96	493 (5.9)	207	286	58.0
97–112	759 (9.1)	319	440	58.0
113–128	498 (5.9)	198	300	60.2
129–144	301 (3.6)	102	199	66.1
145–160	392 (4.7)	140	252	64.3
161–176	170 (2.0)	40	130	76.5
177–192	124 (1.5)	40	84	67.7
193+	444 (5.3)	143	301	67.8
Column Total	8,386 (100.0)	5,448 (65.0)	2,938 (35.0)	

*Percentage figures are in parenthesis.

†Terminations include only those 1973 BRP rehabilitants with an MBR and an R 300 record with appropriate entries for the variables used who left the DI beneficiary rolls because of recovery for any duration during the period July 1972 to January 1977.

Source: 1973 SRS-RSA R 300 Tape and SSA Master Beneficiary Record.

those rehabilitated at these higher wages not terminate? Some individuals may have discovered they were not capable of sustaining work effort for long durations and were forced to leave their jobs. Others may have decided to alter their labor market behavior so as to continue to receive benefits.

Although the legal test depends upon SGA levels, individuals must be aware that jobs with precarious tenure at low wage rates may not be preferable to receipt of DI benefits. The wage is the wage at closure as recorded by the counselor, and the benefit is the total family benefit actually received by the individual. We have not made adjustments for the fact that benefits are tax free, whereas the worker must pay social security taxes and income taxes on wages he earns. An additional consideration is that receipt of DI benefits brings with it the opportunity for leisure and eliminates the various expenses associated with work such as travel costs, special clothes, and extra expenditures for food.

In Table 1-12 we consider the reported wage divided by the actual benefit to arrive at a wage-benefit ratio. It can be seen from Table 1-12 that termination rates increase with increases in the wage-benefit ratio. Termination rates are comparatively low when wage-benefit ratios were less than one. If the rehabilitant's wage-benefit ratio is less than one, even though his closure wage may be higher than SGA, the probability of his terminating is less than 25 percent. Significantly, once the wage-benefit ratio equals or exceeds one, the rate of termination doubles to approximately 50 percent or higher. Perhaps the reality of rehabilitating DI beneficiaries is that they must be closed at a wage which is not only greater than the SGA level but also equal to or greater than their monthly benefit payments. The counselor who fails to close out cases at wages comparable to benefit levels may be fighting a losing battle if the objective is termination and eventual savings to the trust fund. We can best assess the relative importance of the wage-benefit ratio if we discuss it together with the several demographic characteristics of the client.

Table 1-12 Wage/Benefit Ratio and the Rate of Termination

Wage/Benefit Ratio	Category Total*	Nonterminations	Terminations†	Rate of Terminations
0.00–0.25	2,342 (27.9)	2,239	103	4.4
0.26–0.50	525 (6.3)	452	73	13.9
0.51–0.75	463 (5.5)	360	103	22.2
0.76–1.00	513 (6.1)	305	208	40.5
1.01–1.25	511 (6.1)	252	259	50.7
1.26–1.50	506 (6.0)	235	271	53.6
1.51–1.75	468 (5.6)	179	289	61.8
1.76–2.00	365 (4.4)	129	236	64.7
Greater than 2.00	1,653 (19.7)	503	1,150	69.6
Insufficient data	1,040 (12.4)	794	246	23.7
Column Total:	8,386 (100.0)	5,448 (65.0)	2,938 (35.0)	

*Percentage figures are in parenthesis.

† Terminations include only those 1973 BRP rehabilitants with both an MBR and a R 300 record with appropriate entries for the variables used who left the DI beneficiary rolls because of recovery for any duration during the period July 1972 to January 1977.

Source: 1973 SRS-RSA R 300 Tape and SSA Master Beneficiary Record.

Probability of Termination Regression Model

At this juncture, we use regression analysis to test the effect of demograhpic and educational factors and the wage-benefit ratios on the probability that a rehabilitated DI beneficiary will terminate. Given the type of model utilized, we are able to interpret the coefficients of each of the independent variables.[22] The results are presented in Table 1-13.

An example will indicate how these results can be used. If a person is a white male BRP rehabilitant and married, and three years had elapsed from onset to closure, and he was in the rehabilitation process for 10 months, and his wage-benefit ratio is one, then the probability of his terminating from the DI rolls would be 42 percent.[23]

If, in our example, the rehabilitant is older, say between 55 and 64, we would subtract from the 42 percent the absolute value of the coefficient for the 55 to 64 age group that is 21 percent. Thus, the rehabilitant in the oldest age group with these same characteristics has only a 21 percent chance of terminating.

If the client is 30 years of age rather than in the 35 to 44 group, the chances of his terminating increase by 9 percent. Thus the probability of his leaving the rolls increases from 42 percent to 51 percent.

The various education variables can be interpreted in a similar fashion. If the rehabilitant is a high school graduate rather than a grade school dropout, the chances of his terminating increase by 8 percent; being single rather than married decreases the probability. The condition classification as usual is difficult to interpret, but orthopedic impairments tend to increase the probability while sensory deprivation and mental disabilities lower the probability.

Our regression model includes two time or duration variables. We measure the number of years from onset of disability to closure. The sign of the variable is negative. For each year, the probability of termination declines but not by a great deal.

Another duration variable is the number of months in re-

Table 1-13 Probability of Termination Regression Results White Male Cohort of 1973 BRP Rehabilitants*

Variable	B Coefficient (Standard Error)	F-Value
Constant†	0.2943713	
55–64 yrs	−0.2059296 (0.02135)	93.033
45–54 yrs	−0.0809262 (0.01687)	23.024
25–34 yrs	0.0875841 (0.01745)	25.205
14–24 yrs	0.1078082 (0.02188)	24.270
College degree	0.0710894 (0.03642)	3.809
1–3 yrs of college	0.0325701 (0.02602)	1.557
High school graduate	0.0768176 (0.01981)	15.038
1–3 yrs of high school	0.0143431 (0.02068)	0.481
8 yrs of elementary school	−0.0056515 (0.02365)	0.057
Married	0.0492536 (0.01489)	10.947
Visual impairment	−0.0856049 (0.02339)	13.390
Hearing impairment	−0.0962519 (0.04397)	4.791
Orthopedic impairment	0.0281692 (0.01632)	2.979
Amputation	0.0067204 (0.02748)	0.060
Mental disorder	−0.0854813 (0.02339)	13.357
Mental retardation	−0.0468561 (0.04885)	0.920
Years from onset to closure	−0.0064693 (0.00044)	212.331
Months from referral to closure	−0.0011450 (0.00032)	12.841
Wage/benefit ratio	0.1083091 (0.00392)	764.962

*Terminations include only those 1973 BRP rehabilitants with both an MBR and an R 300 record with appropriate entries for the variables used who left the DI beneficiary rolls because of recovery for any duration during the period July 1972 to January 1977.

†The constant captures the combined effect of three nonspecified dummy variables in the probability of termination. The variables are age 35–44, 0–7 years of elementary school, and the disability classification for which the etiology is not known or not appropriate.

habilitation status. This variable may provide a rough indication of the severity of disability, although we recognize that certain persons with relatively mild disabilities may be undergoing training programs of relatively long duration. The average number of months in the program is 25 but the standard deviation is 19.5. Obviously, some persons remain in the program only a short time while others, probably undergoing training, extend their period of rehabilitation well beyond the two-year average.

The wage-benefit ratio coefficient is 0.11, indicating that a large change in the wage-benefit ratio from, for example, 1 to 2 would increase the probability of termination by only 11 percent. Would a change from say a wage-benefit ratio of ½ to 1 increase the probability of termination by only 5 percent or 6 percent? The data suggest that the answer would probably be no. Moving up to a wage-benefit ratio of 1 is much more important to the likelihood of termination than increases in the ratio beyond one.

The difficulty with the regression used for Table 1-13 is that it implies a linear relationship between the probability of termination and wage-benefit ratio. Such a relationship does not appear to be the case. To overcome the difficulty, we subdivided the sample into those receiving a closure wage less than their benefits and those receiving a closure wage equal to or greater than their benefit levels. The results of the regression are presented in Table 1-14.

It can be seen from the table that the significance and explanatory power of the variables change. In fact, there is a statistically significant structural shift of the regression line around the wage-benefit ratio of one.

The most significant change is in reference to the wage-benefit ratio itself. Increases in the wage-benefit ratio up to a value of one improve greatly the chances that an individual will terminate, but beyond that level, further improvement in the wage-benefit ratio have a much smaller effect.

In an attempt to examine the role of the SGA limit, we ran

Table 1-14 Probability of Termination Regression Results White Male Cohort of 1973 BRP Rehabilitants*

Variable	Those with Wage/Benefit Ratios of Less Than One B Coefficient (Standard Error)	F-Value	Those with Wage/Benefit Ratios Equal to or Greater Than One B Coefficient (Standard Error)	F-Value
Constant†	0.0798911		0.5213107	
55–64 yrs	−0.0976900 (0.02063)	22.433	−0.2204099 (0.03731)	34.907
45–54 yrs	−0.0581019 (0.01762)	10.868	−0.0453020 (0.02547)	3.162
25–34 yrs	0.0702263 (0.01965)	12.773	0.0389751 (0.02471)	2.482
14–24 yrs	0.0575174 (0.02864)	4.034	0.1034945 (0.02875)	12.959
College degree	0.0976933 (0.03949)	6.120	0.0638810 (0.05345)	1.429
1–3 yrs of college	−0.0459096 (0.02904)	2.499	0.0736811 (0.03801)	3.758
High school graduate	0.0211751 (0.02024)	1.094	0.0956540 (0.03106)	9.485
1–3 yrs of high school	−0.0255230 (0.02102)	1.474	0.0445341 (0.03255)	1.872
8 yrs of elementary school	−0.0086072 (0.02359)	0.133	0.0147545 (0.03771)	0.153
Married	0.0518518 (0.01688)	9.431	0.0831776 (0.02081)	15.969
Visual impairment	−0.0790213 (0.02404)	10.805	−0.0521420 (0.03605)	2.092
Hearing impairment	−0.0631094 (0.04669)	1.827	−0.0998160 (0.06506)	2.354
Orthopedic impairment	0.0204427 (0.01965)	1.341	0.0565990 (0.02371)	5.696
Amputation	−0.0067797 (0.02909)	0.054	0.0658036 (0.04092)	2.586
Mental disorder	−0.0455479 (0.02507)	3.300	−0.0985053 (0.03433)	8.233
Mental retardation	−0.0661832 (0.04752)	1.940	−0.1088044 (0.08300)	1.718
Years from onset to closure	−0.0031035 (0.00046)	45.468	−0.0097732 (0.00069)	201.884
Months from referral to closure	−0.0012636 (0.00035)	12.827	0.0026601 (0.00046)	0.337
Wage/benefit ratio	0.4333570 (0.01993)	472.740	0.0236662 (0.00534)	19.677

*Terminations include only those 1973 BRP rehabilitants with both an MBR and an R 300 record with appropriate entries for the variables used who left the DI beneficiary rolls because of recovery for any duration during the period July 1972 to January 1973.

†The constant captures the combined effect of three nonspecified dummy variables in the probability of termination. Those variables are: age 35–44, 0–7 years of elementary school, and the disability classification for which the etiology is not known or not appropriate.

similar regressions on those rehabilitants with a recorded weekly wage at closure of $46 or more so that everyone in the sample is a potential terminee.

The results of those regressions are presented in Table 1-15. In the case of individuals who are earning more than the SGA limit but whose benefits exceed earnings, only a few factors significantly affect the probability of termination. Of the statistically significant factors, however, the wage-benefit ratio again has the greatest effect on the probability of termination, regardless of the level of benefits or earnings.

Our finding, that the wage-benefit ratio has a significant effect on the probability of termination, suggests that there are certain disincentives to terminate in the system which persuade some beneficiaries to remain on the rolls because their economic position is better. While it is not feasible to do an extended empirical analysis of the disincentive effect of each of the provisions of the DI program, we are able to use these findings in the following discussion of some provisions and proposed changes in the DI program.

Disincentives and the SGA Limit

Within the DI program there is a continuum of disability cases extending from the diaried cases, who are likely to recover medically after some period of time, to the most severely disabled, who are incapable of any work effort outside of the home. In between these two extremes are individuals with varying degrees of ability to participate in the labor force. The question of disincentives concerns the DI beneficiaries in this middle range who have a choice between labor and leisure.

The sample of FY 1973 rehabilitants we have been using have been rehabilitated and have demonstrated an ability to work at a job for at least 60 days. Therefore, this sample does fall into a group for which the question of disincentives is relevant. Any evidence we have of the existence of work disincentives is derived from the empirical findings for this select group of DI beneficiaries.

Table 1-15 Probability of Termination Regression Results White Male Cohort of 1973 BRP Rehabilitants with Wages at Closure Equal to or Greater than the 1974 SGA Limit*

Variable	Those with Wage/Benefit Ratios of Less Than One B Coefficient (Standard Error)	F-Value	Those with Wage/Benefit Ratios Equal to or Greater Than One B Coefficient (Standard Error)	F-Value
Constant†	0.4300537		0.5814991	
55–64 yrs	−0.2854122 (0.09620)	8.803	−0.2144637 (0.03857)	30.910
45–54 yrs	−0.1525818 (0.06372)	5.733	−0.0470364 (0.025484)	3.313
25–34 yrs	0.0691308 (0.05625)	1.510	0.03231303 (0.02510)	1.656
14–24 yrs	−0.0442063 (0.08530)	0.269	0.1018093 (0.02936)	12.023
College degree	—	—	0.0474723 (0.05060)	0.880
1–3 yrs of college	−0.1442921 (0.09326)	2.394	0.0474631 (0.03346)	2.012
High school graduate	0.0114146 (0.06775)	0.028	0.0617962 (0.02482)	6.198
1–3 yrs of high school	−0.1581033 (0.07265)	4.735	0.0143625 (0.02678)	0.288
8 yrs of elementary school	−0.0549270 (0.09112)	0.363	—	—
Married	0.0407135 (0.06263)	0.423	0.0702262 (0.02124)	10.936
Visual impairment	−0.1356544 (0.09072)	2.236	−0.0566810 (0.03686)	2.365
Hearing impairment	0.1680923 (0.21096)	0.635	−0.1090723 (0.06789)	2.581
Orthopedic impairment	0.1471014 (0.05929)	6.155	0.0559578 (0.02404)	5.417
Amputation	0.1219033 (0.12219)	0.995	0.0600825 (0.04132)	2.114
Mental disorder	0.096286 (0.08362)	1.326	−0.1006424 (0.03509)	8.228
Mental retardation	−0.1190880 (0.19520)	0.372	−0.1398038 (0.09147)	2.336
Years from onset to closure	−0.0075531 (0.00160)	22.263	−0.0100812 (0.00076)	174.978
Months from referral to closure	−0.0041522 (0.00128)	10.488	0.0004472 (0.00047)	0.911
Wage/benefit ratio	0.3113334 (0.13884)	5.029	0.0186344 (0.00537)	12.056

*Terminations include only those 1973 BRP rehabilitants with both an MBR and an R 300 record with appropriate entries for the variables used who left the DI beneficiary rolls because of recovery during the period July 1972 to January 1977.

†The constant captures the combined effect of three nonspecified dummy variables in the probability of termination. Those variables are: age 35–44, 0–7 years of elementary school, and the disability classification for which the etiology is not known or not appropriate.

One of the elements of the DI program that may create work disincentives and discourage termination is the SGA limit. The SGA limit serves two related purposes. First, it is used to help determine who is eligible for DI benefits. To be awarded benefits, a person with a medical impairment must be incapable of substantial gainful activity. The monthly SGA limit was $200 in 1974. It has been raised periodically and in 1980 was $300.

The second function of the SGA provision is to distinguish DI beneficiaries who are continuing disability cases from those who are not. Once on the DI rolls, a person may undertake trial work for a period of nine months. A month of trial work is now defined as one in which monthly earnings are above $50. Significantly, no maximum earnings level is specified; for the duration of the nine-month period, the person's earnings are not constrained. Beyond the ninth month, however, a person whose earnings exceed the SGA limit is no longer considered disabled. In this way, the SGA limit serves as a simple cut-off mechanism to determine who will continue to receive benefits and who will be terminated from the DI rolls.

The reliance upon a fixed earnings limit in disability determinations poses a number of problems. It may lead to seemingly arbitrary determinations, so that a person earning slightly less than SGA continues to receive benefits, whereas someone earning slightly more than the SGA limit receives no benefits. The worker whose earnings exceed the SGA limit in the month following the trial work period suffers a substantial drop in income when his benefits are terminated. In fact, in that month, if his wages are less than the amount he received in benefits, he faces, in effect, a tax rate of over 100 percent on his income.

For example, assume an individual receives a monthly DI benefit of $325 and is able to earn an additional $270 in wages, after taxes. His total net monthly income during the trial work period is $595, but after the work period his disposable income will fall by $325, amounting to an average tax rate of over 120 percent. The drop in income, together with the loss of Medicare coverage constitute a severe price to pay for the beneficiary uncertain of the success of his return to the labor market. It is understandable, under these conditions, that some beneficiaries may be reluctant to leave the rolls.

It is difficult to specify empirically the aggregate disincentive effects of the SGA limit. Nevertheless, the FY 1973 data on the earnings of recipients do provide some evidence concerning this effect. We know that in 1976, 24.4 percent of the BRP rehabilitants who had not terminated as of January 1977 participated to some degree in the labor market. It is this group of individuals, with their double status as wage earners and beneficiaries, who are of particular interest. The fact that they have shown themselves capable of some labor force participation invites us to ask why they had not terminated. Two explanations are possible: (1) the extent of their impairment made them incapable of earning more than the SGA amount, or (2) they were capable of earning more than the SGA amount, but reasoned that they would suffer a net loss of income if they did so.

In order to reach some conclusion as to whether some individuals do, in fact, fall into this second group, we would have to know something about the productive capacity of the nonterminees. The best measure of their capacity available to us is their wage at closure. Most rehabilitants have only begun their trial work period at the time of closure; therefore, at this point in time, they are not under any constraints to limit their income, and their earnings at time of rehabilitation are an accurate reflection of their true earnings capacity. We can reasonably conclude, then, that those nonterminees who earned a wage at closure that was under the SGA, would not likely be voluntarily restricting their earnings in subsequent years to avoid exceeding the SGA limit. The statistics bear this out: Of the 3,667 non-terminated rehabilitants closed at a wage less than the 1974 SGA figure ($200 a month), only 519, or less than 15 percent, had any earnings in 1976.[24]

Since earnings of less than $200 a month would not have resulted in any benefit reduction, it would appear that most of these persons are not working because of the severity of their condition and not due to the disincentive effect of the SGA. While the disincentive effect may have been minimal for the group of people closed at a wage below SGA, it does have clear relevance to those cases where the wage at closure exceeded the SGA. There were 2,394 nonterminated rehabilitants closed at a wage which exceeded $46 a week. Of these, 960, or about 40 percent, were participating in the labor market to some degree in 1976. We might legitimately infer that for some of these persons, the SGA did act as a work disincentive. The data support the hypothesis that some individuals are capable of earning enough income to leave the rolls, but choose instead to use the SGA provision as a limit on the income they earn in order to maintain their benefit status and remain on the rolls.

Because of these suspected disincentives, several proposals have been made to change the SGA limit and the method in which it is used. For example, in arguing for an increase in the SGA limit the GAO claimed the $200 SGA level made the transition difficult for the beneficiary moving from a benefit to a work status.[25] Although raising the SGA limit permits the beneficiary to better gauge the probability of his remaining a permanent participant in the labor force before terminating, any increase most likely has an increased disincentive effect as well, particularly for those marginal cases whose decision to terminate under the old limit would only be reached after some deliberation. The individual who would refuse benefits and choose to depend solely on his or her earnings at an SGA limit of $200, may find it economically advantageous to remain on the DI rolls at higher SGA limits.

We do not dispute the claim that raising the limit may increase the amount of time individual beneficiaries participate in the labor force. In fact, under the SGA limit of $200, a person working 18 to 20 hours a week at the minimum wage was in danger of losing his benefits. The labor markets that are most accessible to the DI beneficiary who is uncertain of his or her ability to sustain a living wage are the secondary labor markets paying low wages and permitting part-time employment. Some individuals may be capable of commanding a higher wage even though they are unable to participate on a full-time basis, but because of the SGA limit they would restrict their participation. We recognize, then, that raising the limit would permit these individuals to participate more fully in accordance with their capabilities.

Our position, however, is that an increase in the SGA limit does not provide incentive to *leave* the rolls. Two qualifications should be mentioned. First, creating the opportunity for some beneficiaries to participate more fully in the labor market without losing their benefits may aid their rehabilitation and provide them with the confidence to eventually terminate. Second, with the experience of greater participation in the labor market, beneficiaries who do eventually terminate may have a lower rate of recidivism. Obviously, both these qualifications are speculative and can only be tested after the higher SGA limit has been in effect for some time. In brief, we conclude that raising the SGA limit probably diminishes the work disincentives for DI beneficiaries but not the disincentives to terminate.

One suggestion for reducing the "notch effect," i.e., the sudden drop in income for terminees who lose all benefits, is to adopt a benefit payment method similar to the retirement test.[26] Earnings above the SGA limit would be taxed at the marginal rate of 50 percent. In this case every two dollars earned over $200 would result in the reductions of benefits by one dollar. For example, a person with no earnings might receive $300 in benefits, but if he earned $300 a month, benefits would be reduced to $250 a month, and if earnings were $500 a month, the monthly benefit would be reduced to $150.

Several objections can be raised concerning this proposal. One is that many people who have already terminated might find it worthwhile to reapply for DI status and return to the rolls in order to receive partial benefits while continuing to work. A more fundamental objection, however, is that this method of paying benefits to rehabilitants contradicts the rationale for a DI program. At present, the program is designed to pay benefits on the basis of past earnings to those who have been determined to be totally disabled. If, under this proposal, a person is able to earn over $500 a month and still receive benefits, the whole concept of the program would be changed.

The Trial Work Period

We have seen that the one provision that does allow the DI recipient to work without constraints on his income is the trial work period. During this period, the beneficiary can choose a job paying a wage commensurate with his productive capabilities without fear of losing benefits. One of the purposes of the provision is to enable the beneficiary to determine whether he is capable of sustaining himself through work effort without DI benefits.

The trial work period is designed as an incentive provision and as such cannot be categorized as contributing to the disincentive problem. Changes in trial work provisions could be made, however, that would help to eliminate the disincentives to work and to termination that now exist in the BRP program. One possibility is simply to increase the duration of the trial work period. The assumption underlying such a change is that nine months is too short a time for a valid assessment of the work potential of the beneficiary. While we have little evidence at present that would enable us to evaluate a proposal of this kind, we can speculate on some of the effects of the change. Beneficiaries who terminate would, of course, terminate at a later date. Benefit payments to these individuals over the extended period of trial work would result in an immediate increase in the costs to the trust fund. On the other hand, the longer period of trial work might give beneficiaries greater confidence in their ability to participate in the labor force, and consequently bring about a higher termination rate. In any case, as an alternative to raising the SGA limit, extending the trial work period has this important advantage: it would not act to decrease the number of beneficiaries eventually terminating.

Another proposed change in the trial work period entails increasing the amount one can earn per month. At present, a month in which earnings are $50 or more counts towards the trial work period. Since the purpose of the trial work period is to allow the beneficiary adequate time to assess whether he or she is capable of sustaining her- or himself for longer periods, the $50 limit seems rather low. Valuable months of trial work are used up in earning a level of income that would be unlikely to lead to the termination of benefits. In addition, many beneficiaries, after their trial work period at low wages has expired, lack the assurance that they can sustain participation in the labor force; consequently, they do not risk losing their benefits by seeking out more hours of work or work at a higher wage.

Raising the monthly amount, to the SGA limit of $230 for example, would remedy some of these difficulties by giving the beneficiary an opportunity for a more realistic appraisal of his or her ability to terminate. Therefore, with a higher limit triggering the trial work period, one would expect that beneficiaries might emerge from the trial work experience with greater confidence and better job qualifications. The net effect might be higher rates of termination. In addition, the marginal costs to the program might be fairly low, because few beneficiaries terminate immediately after the end of the trial work period when they have only been earning a little over the $50 limit. In other words, one would not expect terminations to be delayed simply because beneficiaries can earn more (but not more than the SGA limit) before the trial work period is triggered.

DI Benefit Levels

The benefit formula is designed to provide the low-income worker with a higher primary insurance benefit relative to past earnings. This redistribution effect is somewhat offset, however, by the family maximum limits. A 1.5 family maximum limit is applied to individuals with the lowest average monthly income, increases to 1.88 for those with average monthly earnings of approximately $450, and falls only slightly to 1.75 for the remainder of the benefit table for individuals with average earnings of $1,000 or more per month.

There has been some concern that the current high level of benefits discourages those who are able to work from terminating. The suggestions for reform have included reducing the PIA or the family maximum limits.

An estimate of the incentive effect resulting from reducing benefits can be derived from the regression results for the probability of termination model. As we mentioned earlier, the coefficients can be used to predict what incremental impact a change in the value of a variable, such as the benefit amount, will have on the probability of termination.[27] We find that a 10-percent decrease in benefits will increase the probability of termination by 0.024 if the initial ratio of wage to benefits is 0.8 (Table 1-15).[28] The closer the relationship of wages to benefits, the greater the incentive effect from a 10-percent reduction in benefits. Reduced benefits, however, will have less of an incentive as the wage-benefit ratio increases.

Although a reduction in benefits may induce some individuals to leave the rolls, other beneficiaries, particularly those with severe functional limitations, may be precluded from engaging in work for any extended period of time. Unless these individuals can be identified, lowering benefits to increase incentives for some will entail penalizing others who are incapable of substantial gainful activity because of their disabling condition.

There is not only concern over high benefit levels but also over the age-distribution of benefits. There is an apparent inequity between younger and older workers in terms of the benefits received and the percent of past earnings that the benefits replace. In the public hearings on the DI program[29] the following hypothetical example was used. Assume that a father age 55 and his son age 25 were employed throughout their working lives at the maximum taxable wage under social security, and that both became disabled in February of 1976. The son would be entitled to a primary benefit of $515 a month (maximum family benefit of $901.60) while the father would be entitled to a primary benefit of $356.60 a month (maximum family benefit of $639.40). Since the earnings of father and son were the same just prior to onset, the benefit going to the younger worker replaces a greater percentage of past earnings. The equity question depends in part on what policymakers regard as the proper measure for earnings. Should the measure be a person's earnings just prior to onset, or an estimate of the level of income that the person would have earned had he not become disabled?

The high replacement rate for the young based upon prior earnings is not only cited as evidence of the inequitable distribution of benefits but also as evidence of a rather severe disincentive effect for the younger worker to return to work.

Replacement Rates

Many factors influence the probability of termination, and the data we are using only identify a sample from all the DI beneficiaries, namely, those rehabilitated in FY 73. To investigate the issue of the relationship between prior earnings, benefits and termination in greater depth we have estimated replacement rates for the group of FY 73 rehabilitants. The replacement rate measures the ratio of benefits received at closure to the earnings received two years prior to the onset of disability, indexed (at 5 percent per annum) to the time of closure.

Table 1-16 shows the termination rates for each replacement rate category by age categories.[30] As we expected, the data show varying replacement rates for the different age categories. Of those rehabilitants with earnings, 52.6 percent and 61 percent in the respective age categories 14 to 24 and 25 to 34 had replacement ratios of less than 0.5, compared with 68.6 percent, 73.3 percent and 79.1 percent for the age categories 35 to 44, 45 to 54 and 55 to 64. In other words, in reading down each column of Table 1-16, we find that the older the worker, the lower the replacement rate.

Table 1-16 Replacement Rates (rr) and Rates of Termination by Age Categories

Age Categories	(No earnings)	0 rr .25†	0.25 rr 0.5	0.5 rr 0.75	0.75 rr 1.0	rr 1.0
14–24						
Rehabs	40	175	321	108	57	77
% of total	(4.2)	(18.6)	(34.0)	(11.5)	(6.0)	(8.2)
Terminations	4	97	224	68	34	38
Rate*	(10.0)	(55.5)	(69.8)	(63.0)	(59.6)	(49.4)
25–34						
Rehabs	40	515	580	161	50	161
% of total	(2.2)	(28.7)	(32.3)	(9.0)	(2.8)	(9.0)
Terminations	10	227	310	78	26	95
Rate	(25.0)	(44.1)	(53.4)	(48.4)	(52.0)	(59.0)
35–44						
Rehabs	67	809	574	109	67	123
% of total	(3.3)	(40.1)	(25.5)	(5.4)	(3.3)	(6.1)
Terminations	20	292	264	54	32	80
Rate	(29.9)	(36.1)	(46.0)	(49.5)	(47.8)	(65.0)
45–54						
Rehabs	55	907	511	111	48	115
% of total	(2.8)	(46.9)	(26.4)	(5.7)	(2.5)	(5.9)
Terminations	15	252	163	50	27	76
Rate	(27.3)	(27.8)	(31.9)	(45.0)	(56.3)	(66.1)
55–65						
Rehabs	29	498	221	37	17	48
% of total	(3.2)	(54.8)	(24.3)	(4.1)	(1.9)	(5.3)
Terminations	2	62	25	9	6	22
Rate	(6.9)	(12.4)	(11.3)	(24.3)	(35.3)	(45.8)

*Terminations include only those 1973 BRP rehabilitants who 1) had both an MBR and an R 300 record with appropriate entries for the variables used, and 2) left the DI beneficiary rolls because of recovery during the period July 1972 to January 1977. The recovery might be of any duration. Excluded are those whose benefits were terminated due to death.

†Replacement rates were computed in the following manner: $rr = \dfrac{\text{benefit at closure} \times 12}{\text{Earn}(t-1) + \text{Earn}(t-2)} \times (1.05)^n$ where t = the year of onset and n is the time from onset to closure given that T is 1962.

Source: SRS-RSA 1973 R 300 Tape and SSA Earnings and Master Beneficiary Records.

We would also expect, at first glance, that each increase in the replacement rate would produce a decrease in the termination rate. Such a finding would lend support to the argument that high benefit levels relative to prior earnings act as disincentives to terminate. But as we read across the rows, for example, the 35 to 44 age category row, we see that the percentage of those terminating increases as the replacement rates increase. There are, however, a number of explanations for the apparent anomaly that an increase in benefits relative to prior earnings lead to an increase in the rates of termination. First, those rehabilitated beneficiaries with high replacement rates are young and more likely than the older beneficiaries to be married, to have growing families, and to receive close to the maximum family benefits. Their growing family responsibilities probably act as powerful incentive for them to return to the labor market.

Second, the sample is drawn from those beneficiaries who have been rehabilitated. It can be expected that the stock of human capital has been increased for the young who were low wage earners prior to onset, with the result that their new earnings potential may be significantly greater. In other words, the effect of a better education may have increased the probability of termination for those with low earnings prior to onset to such a degree that it cancels out any disincentive arising from a high replacement rate.

Although we could introduce the two explanatory variables identified above, family status and education, into a regression that includes replacement rates and termination rates, there would be diminishing returns as the calculations based on our sample data became more complex. This is because the most significant explanation of the results from Table 1-16 is probably the fact that replacement rates had little or no effect on the decisions to terminate by those in our sample group. The rehabilitants that make up the group had undoubtedly been out of the labor market for two or more years prior to the closure of their cases; it is probable that even more time had elapsed before termination. We have indexed the predisability wages for changes in the general wage level (by 5 percent per year), but we have not taken into account the stage of each beneficiary's life cycle or the age-earning profile at the time of the onset of disability. The replacement rate may not be as meaningful, therefore, as the wage-benefit ratio, despite the difficulties that exist in using the beneficiary's wage at closure as a gauge of his value in the labor force. Replacement rates may be most useful in determining the disincentive effects of participating in the labor force or going on the rolls at the time of onset of disability. They may be less relevant for determining whether someone terminates or not.

Conclusion

Overall the regression results suggest that the obvious method for reducing work and termination disincentives is to increase the wage-benefit ratio. Although this could be achieved by lowering benefits, we reject that option on equity grounds. Improving the wages of beneficiaries can be achieved by liberalizing the provisions of the trial work period, by improving the performance of rehabilitation counselors and by the long-term strategy of making the labor market more amenable to the rehabilitated population. Such a strategy could be implemented in two ways: first, by selection and rehabilitation of those DI beneficiaries with the greatest probability of termination; and second, by strong enforcement of sections 503 and 504 of the Rehabilitation Act of 1973, which require affirmative action and nondiscrimination in the employment of the handicapped.

The BRP is the only program with the avowed objective of terminating beneficiaries from the DI rolls. It has been in existence for a little over ten years. One can look at the past decade as a kind of experimental period in which the BRP has demonstrated it can terminate beneficiaries without loss to the DI trust fund. The evidence points to the fact that the BRP saves the trust fund money, in addition to providing significant nonpecuniary benefits to its clients as well.

It is our contention that the program can be adjusted to be

even more efficient. The adjustments we recommend include reforms in the program's management, financing and monitoring. A central unit within SSA should be solely responsible for BRP activities. A management information system should be developed to produce accurate data on the program's performance. Data should be fed back to the counselor level to improve the efficiency of the selection criteria. A financing scheme based upon savings to the trust fund and state-by-state results should be implemented to assure the independence and solvency of the program. Finally, further research, in the form of experiments, should be conducted to identify ways and means of increasing the rate of termination of DI beneficiaries. Implementation of these recommendations should bring about the maturation of the BRP into an even more productive feature of the DI system.

A Postscript

Since our study was completed, two significant developments in rehabilitation policy have occurred: the Rehabilitation Services Administration has changed its formula for allocating special funds to the states and Congress changed some features of the DI program and the Beneficiary Rehabilitation Program when it passed the "Social Security Disability Amendments of 1980."

Beginning in Fiscal Year 1980, RSA is allocating special program funds on the basis of relative state performance in achieving rehabilitations at SGA. As RSA noted, "The use of SGA rehabilitations as a measure of an agency's performance, more than ever before, places the funding incentive closer to the rehabilitation effort and acts as a clear-cut reward for successful rehabilitation."[31] Using data for 1978, adjusted to account for differences in the SGA level for blind and nonblind recipients, RSA recalculated state allotments. Even though states were protected somewhat by a rule limiting any reduction to one-third of its 1979 allotment, the new formula produced some substantial differences in comparisons to the 1979 allotments. For instance in the BRP, 13 states and Puerto Rico were scheduled to receive less than they had been allotted in 1979. New York lost nearly two million dollars and Florida nearly a million. Illinois, Missouri, Texas and Washington were each scheduled to have their allotments increased by over one million dollars.

The real test of the effectiveness of the new formula will occur in the coming years. As states act to win larger budgets (or prevent losing what they have) it will be interesting to watch what happens to SGA rehabilitations and terminations. The new financing formula will help answer questions about the effectiveness of states in altering counselor behavior. Without increases in real spending and without major changes designed to affect client incentives and disincentives, we believe RSA has taken a positive step forward in improving performance in the BRP.

The other side of the performance coin was addressed in recent amendments to the DI program.[32] In fact, Congress had even considered abolishing the special programs, but the idea was discarded, partly in recognition of RSA's change in the funding formula. Nonetheless, Congress acted in other areas in the hope of gaining still more improvements in the rehabilitation of DI recipients.

One feature of the DI program often cited as discouraging rehabilitation was the potential loss of Medicare benefits. The problem was heightened by the requirement of another two year waiting period should the individual again become eligible for DI benefits. The new amendments eliminated the second waiting period for those becoming eligible within 60 months and extended Medicare eligibility for 36 months following the cessation of DI benefits provided that the individual had not medically recovered.

Other changes designed to encourage DI recipients to seek employment included broadening the definition of extraordinary work expenses and extending the trial work period. Congress adjusted the concept of extraordinary work expenses to include costs incurred by the individual for medication and equipment related to the disabling condition. The trial work period was extended to 24 months with no benefits paid during the last 12 months but with automatic reinstatement of benefits if earnings were less than the SGA amount.

Two other changes possibly could have an indirect effect on BRP success. By placing a cap on maximum benefits the amendments will lead to lower benefits for some persons. As a result, there will be a reduced incentive to apply for or maintain beneficiary status. Congress also established authority to waive benefits and Medicare provisions in order to allow experiments to uncover methods to encourage people to return to work.

Both the RSA and legislative reforms indicate the strong concern over the costs of disability programs and the failure of rehabilitation programs to do a better job. In light of the findings of our own research and the work of others, these changes seem to be a logical step to improve rehabilitation performance. The reasoning and the research on which they rely will be put to the test in the coming months.

NOTES

1. *Committee Staff Report on the Disability Insurance Program*, Committee on Ways and Means, U.S. House of Representatives (Washington, D.C.: U.S. Government Printing Office, July, 1974, p. 285).
2. Ralph Treitel, "Financing of the Disability Beneficiary Rehabilitation," *Social Security Bulletin*, Vol. 32, No. 4 (April, 1969), p. 30.
3. Ralph Treitel, "Recovery of Disabled After Trust Fund Financing of Rehabilitation," *Social Security Bulletin*, Vol. 36, No. 2 (February 1973), p. 24.
4. The BRP was established "to the end that savings will result to the Trust Fund as a result of rehabilitating the maximum number of such individuals into productive activity." (Social Security Act, Title II, Section 222 (d).)
5. Social Security Act, Title II, Section 222 (d).

6. Comptroller General of the United States, Report to the Congress, *Improvements Needed in Rehabilitating Social Security Disability Insurance Beneficiaries* (Washington, D.C.: Department of Health, Education and Welfare, May 13, 1976, p. 3).
7. *Senate Report*, Calendar No. 389, Rept. 404, Part I, 1965, p. 103.
8. Initial allotment state A = $\frac{\text{\# of DI beneficiaries residing in state A}}{\text{total \# of DI beneficiaries}}$ × total allotment. The initial allotments for FY 1977 were based upon the DI population data for June, 1975. See the postscript for a recent change in the allotment method.
9. Tables M6 and M9, *Social Security Bulletin*, Vol. 40, No. 5 and previous issues; *State Vocational Rehabilitation Agency Program Data*, Department of Health, Education, and Welfare, Washington, D.C., 1974, 1975, 1976 reports and *Financial Plan 1978*; and the GAO Report, p. 5.
10. Table 1 and Table M6, *Social Security Bulletin*, Vol. 40, No. 5. As a percentage of the previous year's total assets BRP allotments grew from 0.48 percent in 1972 to an estimated 1.61 percent in 1978.
11. See Francisco Bayo, "Disability Rehabilitation with Trust Fund Money" (memorandum to Mr. Robert J. Myers, Chief Actuary, SSA, Office of the Actuary), Baltimore, June 10, 1969. Robert J. Myers, "Actuarial Analysis of Disability Beneficiary Rehabilitation Experience" (memorandum to Mr. Robert M. Ball, Commissioner of Social Security), Baltimore, June 13, 1969. Ida C. Merriam, "Disability Beneficiary Rehabilitation Experience" (memorandum to Commissioner Ball), Baltimore, June 27, 1969. Bernard Popick, "Actuarial Analysis of Disability Beneficiary Rehabilitation Experience" (memorandum to Commissioner Ball), Baltimore, October 24, 1969.
12. Rehabilitation Services Paid from Social Security Trust Funds," Office of the Actuary, Social Security, Dec. 1970.
13. A memorandum from Francisco Bayo, Deputy Chief Actuary, to Robert M. Ball, Commissioner of Social Security, "Vocational Rehabilitation with Trust Fund Money" (August 19, 1970).
14. The GAO Report indicates that the estimate was prepared for the Senate Committee on Finance and led SSA to conclude that program funding should be increased. Congress did increase funding to 1.25 percent in FY73 and 1.5 percent in subsequent years. See page 8 of the GAO Report.
15. House of Representatives, Committee on Ways and Means, *Committee Staff Report on the Disability Insurance Program* (Washington, D.C.: U.S. Government Printing Office, 1974, pp. 303–305).

16. These assumptions were provided by the Office of the Actuary staff in a meeting at SSA on June 24, 1976.
17. Comptroller General of the United States, General Accounting Office, Report to the Congress, *Improvements Needed in Rehabilitating Social Security Disability Insurance Beneficiaries* (Washington, D.C.: DHEW, May 1976).
18. GAO Report, p. 14.
19. GAO Report, p. 13.
20. RSA, "The Applicability of Linking Rehabilitation Program Funding to State Agency Performance," p. 2.
21. The figure for Ohio is somewhat in question due to some reporting inconsistencies. The relative rankings do not change drastically regardless of this possible data problem.
22. The model in matrix form is $T = XB + U$, where T and U are matrices of the order $n \times 1$, X is n x $(K+1)$ and B is $(K+1) \times 1$. The dependent variable (T) will take on either of two values: one if the individual terminated following rehabilitation and zero otherwise.

    With a dichotomous dependent variable, we have an additive linear probability function. The results of the regression can be interpreted as the conditional probability that termination will occur given all the Xs. The estimated coefficients can separately be used to predict the incremental impact a certain variable or change in the value of that variable will have on the probability of termination.
23. Constant (29.4 percent) + married (4.9 percent) + years from onset to closure (3 × [-0.6 percent]) + months from referral to closure (10 × [-0.1 percent]) + wage-benefit ratio (1.0 × 10.8 percent) equals 42 percent.
24. Data on wages and participation rates of nonterminated rehabilitants are drawn from SRS-RSA 1973 R-300 Tape, SSA Earnings Records and Master Beneficiary Records.
25. Public Hearings before the Subcommittee on Social Security of the Committee on Ways and Means, *Disability Insurance Program*, House of Representatives, 94th Congress, May 1976, p. 30.
26. Public Hearings before the Subcommittee on Social Security of the Committee on Ways and Means, *Disability Insurance Program*, p. 31.
27. The first two partial derivatives indicate the change in the probability of termination resulting from absolute changes in benefits and wages respectively. Partial derivatives 3 and 4 indicate what impact percentage changes in benefits and wages will have on the probability of termination.

1. $\dfrac{\partial T}{\partial B} = \dfrac{-W}{B} Z \cdot a$

2. $\dfrac{\partial T}{\partial W} = \dfrac{1}{B} \cdot a$

3. $\dfrac{\partial T}{\partial \dfrac{B}{B}} = \dfrac{-W}{B} \cdot a$

4. $\dfrac{\partial T}{\dfrac{\partial W}{W}} = \dfrac{W}{B} \cdot a$

Where T is the probability of termination. W and B are Wages and Benefits respectively $\partial\, a$ is the value of the coefficient for the wage-benefit variable.

28. Partial derivative number 3 is used to estimate the change in the probability of termination.

    Change in the probability of termination =
    $$-(W/B \times a \times \% \, DB)$$
    $$= -(.8 \times .311 \times -.1)$$
    $$= 0.024$$

29. Public Hearings before the Subcommittee on Social Security of the Committee on Ways and Means, *Disability Insurance Program*, pp. 23–24.

30. Replacement rates are computed using gross earnings and therefore underestimate the replacement rates based upon net earnings.

31. U.S. Department of Health, Education and Welfare, Office of Human Development Services, Rehabilitation Services Administration, *Program Instruction*, RSA-PI-80-3. Washington, DC, October 23, 1979.

32. U.S. Congress, House, *Social Security Amendments of 1980*, Report No. 96-944, Conference Report to Accompany H.R. 3236, 96th Congress, 2nd Session, May 13, 1980.

Chapter 2

REHABILITATION, EMPLOYMENT, AND THE DISABLED

Sar Levitan and Robert Taggart

THE VOCATIONAL REHABILITATION SYSTEM

An Overview

Vocational rehabilitation has developed into a major national social commitment over the last decade. Characteristically, growth was achieved by the proliferation and expansion of categorical efforts rather than as a result of an overall rehabilitation strategy. Disabled veterans have been provided compensation since the beginning of the Republic, and rehabilitation services were initiated after World War I. The federal/state vocational rehabilitation program also originated in the 1920s.

This chapter is adapted from the authors' book *Jobs for the Disabled*, published by the John Hopkins University Press in 1977. The research and writing of the original paper was done in 1976. While the data generally refer to rehabilitation prior to implementation of the Rehabilitation Act of 1973, the authors' suggestions and criticisms of vocational rehabilitation are still relevant today.

Administered by states with substantial federal support, this program serves those whose physical or mental handicaps limit work and who are likely to benefit from the receipt of services. Clients range from the most severely disabled to those with only secondary work limitations. While the vocational rehabilitation program has always included public assistance and social insurance recipients among its clients, a supplementary effort was begun in 1965 to rehabilitate disability insurance recipients, and in 1972 to aid blind and disabled public assistance beneficiaries. A broad range of employment and training programs were launched in the 1960s to aid the disadvantaged, including a fairly significant number of disabled. Sheltered workshops are the final major component of the rehabilitation system, providing employment for those who have few options in the competitive labor market, including many of the most disadvantaged participants in the federal/state program. There are other disparate education and training activities of lesser significance such as rehabilitation for workers' compensation claimants and social services for disabled welfare recipients. Also, there is an increasing federal effort to combat employer discrimination against the disabled, though it is too early to assess the degree of commitment or the likely impact.

Expansion has been rapid on all fronts in the last decade. In FY 1975, rehabilitation programs served 1.8 million persons, nearly triple the figure a decade earlier (Table 2-1). Expenditures rose over this period from $262 million to $1.7 billion, or 3.7 times, after adjusting for the cost of living increases. During the decade ending in 1975, the federal/state system closed a total of 4 million cases, covering an estimated 3½ million different persons after adjusting for repeaters. Sheltered workshops employed perhaps nearly a million separate clients over the decade, while manpower and veterans programs together reached about half a million handicapped.

Since the disabled may participate in more than one program, these totals exceed the number of separate individuals served. Recipient surveys are one means to assess the degree of

Table 2-1 Vocational Rehabilitation Activity: 1965 and 1975

	Clients Served (thousands)	
	Fiscal 1975	Fiscal 1965
Federal/state vocational rehabilitation		
Basic program	1,143	441
Services for DI recipients	76	—
Services for SSI beneficiaries	46	—
Veterans vocational rehabilitation	27	9
Sheltered workshops	410	150
Manpower programs	135	16
Total	1,837	616

	Public Expenditures (millions)	
Federal/state vocational rehabilitation		
Basic program	869	161
Services for DI recipients	81	—
Services for SSI beneficiaries	48	—
Innovation and expenditures	24	21
Veterans vocational rehabilitation	85*	7*
Sheltered workshops	455	50
Manpower programs	178	23
Total	$1,740	$262

*Does not include special benefits for housing adaptations, cars, or special equipment, or medical and other treatments provided to disabled veterans outside or instead of vocational training; does include estimate of costs of counseling psychologists and vocational rehabilitation specialists employed by the Veterans Administration.

Sources: Manpower Report of the President, 1976 and 1966; William H. Button, "Sheltered Workshops in the United States: An Institutional Overview," *Rehabilitation, Sheltered Workshops and the Disadvantaged* (Ithaca, NY: Cornell University, 1970); *State Vocational Rehabilitation Agency Program Data*, Fiscal Years 1968 and 1975 (Washington: Department of Health, Education and Welfare, 1969, 1976); *Veterans Benefits Under Current Educational Programs* (Washington: Veterans Administration, June 1974); *Caseload Statistics, State Vocational Rehabilitation Agencies, 1974* (Washington: Department of Health, Education and Welfare, 1975); Sar Levitan and Garth Mangum, *Federal Training and Work Programs in the Sixties* (Ann Arbor, Mich.: Institute of Labor and Industrial Relations, 1969); *Annual Report, Administration of Veterans Affairs, 1965* (Washington: Government Printing Office, 1965); Greenleigh Associates, *The Role of Sheltered Workshops in the Rehabilitation of the Severely Handicapped*, (New York: Greenleigh Associates, 1976), Vol. II; *Special Analysis J, Budget of the United States Government, 1977* (Washington, D.C.: U.S. Government Printing Office, January 1976); *Committee Staff Report on the Disability Insurance Program*, House Committee on Ways and Means (Washington: Government Printing Office, July 1974).

double counting and the extensiveness of services. Of course, some biases do exist. Some clients forget or choose to ignore assistance; others may credit only one agency with providing or delivering services when, in fact, several were involved. Yet recognizing these biases, the views of recipients are useful in discounting inflated program data.

A fourth of disabled persons in 1972 reported having received rehabilitation services, and 36 percent of these received them in the prior year (Table 2-2). The likelihood of participation did not vary with the degree of disability, but disabled males were half again as likely to be served as disabled females. More

Table 2-2 Disabled Reporting Having Received Rehabilitation Services, 1966 and 1972

	Ever Received (Thousands)	Percent of Disabled Who had Received Services	Received in Previous Year (Thousands)	Percent of Disabled Who had Received Services in Previous Year
1966				
All disabled	2,136	12	694	4
Severely disabled	802	13	319	5
Occupationally disabled	657	13	173	4
Secondary work limitations	678	10	203	3
1972				
All disabled	3,896	25	1,392	9
Severely disabled	1,914	25	728	9
Occupationally disabled	928	27	305	9
Secondary work limitations	1,054	24	359	8

Source: U.S. Department of Health, Education and Welfare, Social Security Administration, 1966 and 1972 surveys of the disabled, unpublished tabulations.

detailed 1966 data revealed that those under 45 years were twice as likely to have been assisted as those who were older. Recipients of income support were served twice as frequently as other disabled.

Private agencies provide most rehabilitation services. Only a seventh of the currently disabled who had received services listed the federal/state vocational rehabilitation program as the provider. One in ten reported assistance directly from the Veterans Administration. Altogether, one-third received services from any public agency. Personal physicians provided services to more than a fifth, and a hospital or rehabilitation center to more than two-fifths (Table 2-3). The secondary role of public agencies as service providers is perhaps not startling, since they frequently contract with private deliverers rather than providing aid directly. Yet only a third of disabled recipients reported that services were arranged by public agencies. Doctors and the disabled themselves assumed primary responsibility.

Three-fourths of the disabled who had received rehabilitation services felt that the services had helped in some way, such as improving mobility, self-care capacity, self-confidence, or employability. Yet only 11 percent claimed they got a job or a better job as a result, and only 8 percent that they were enabled to do their old job better. Less than one in eight severely disabled recipients felt that rehabilitation contributed to labor market success.

These data raise some important issues. First, there is a vast disparity between activity levels reported by program officials and by the disabled. Only 1.4 million disabled persons in 1972 and 335,000 recoverees claimed they received services from any source in the prior year. If 11 percent of services were arranged by vocational rehabilitation agencies, 6 percent by public welfare agencies, 10 percent by the Veterans Administration, and 7 percent by other public agencies, an estimated 600,000 persons would have received services arranged by public agencies. Yet in fiscal 1972 the vocational rehabilitation program alone reported serving 1.1 million cases, while man-

Table 2-3 Source of Rehabilitation Services Received by Disabled, 1972

	\multicolumn{3}{c}{Percent of Persons Reporting Services*}
	Disabled	Severely Disabled	Recovered
Service Provider			
Vocational rehabilitation agency	13.9	10.9	6.6
Veterans Administration	10.2	10.1	11.9
Public welfare	6.2	6.0	.8
Other public	9.1	8.8	7.4
Hospital or rehabilitation center	43.5	47.2	46.8
School	6.8	3.9	5.5
Own doctor	21.0	21.4	26.9
Other private person	5.3	6.2	3.8
Employer (on the job)	6.0	3.5	11.6
Private agency	5.9	6.2	6.8
Not available	1.6	2.5	1.1
Arranger of Services			
Vocational rehabilitation agency	10.6	9.4	4.4
Veterans Administration	10.2	10.3	12.7
Public welfare	6.1	5.9	1.1
Other public	6.5	7.3	6.6
Own doctor	51.0	55.3	57.0
Other private person	4.3	4.2	1.5
Employer	6.7	4.2	10.2
Private agency	2.1	2.3	5.3
Disabled individual	15.1	14.8	18.8
Not available	1.5	.8	2.2

*Some report more than one source of services.

Source: U.S. Department of Health, Education and Welfare, Social Security Administration, 1972 Survey of the Disabled, unpublished tabulations.

power and veterans programs assisted an estimated 100,000 and sheltered workshops another 300,000. Some clients might not have known which agency arranged their services, or even that any public agency was involved. Clients might not have credited services received if they involved only light counseling or placement, but this only suggests that the services did not have much impact. Differences of this magnitude are difficult to reconcile.

It is also difficult to reconcile the performance claims of rehabilitation programs with impact assessments of the disabled. In FY 1972 some 300,000 persons were reportedly placed in jobs, not counting placements by the manpower and veterans programs. Yet only a fourth of the disabled who had ever received rehabilitation services from any source believed that these improved their status in the labor market. And if this held true for the 600,000 persons receiving services arranged by public agencies in 1971, then the total aided by *all* public programs in improving employability would be only 150,000, or half of the annual number reported successfully placed by the vocational rehabilitation program alone.

These aggregate survey data are not fully conclusive, but they offer a striking and useful contrast to the more extensive programmatic data that usually serve as the basis for analysis. For instance, program data can leave the impression that public efforts are the major source of rehabilitation services. This is not the case. Survey information raises questions about the extent of double-counting in the agency reported data, and the degree to which meaningful services are provided. It also suggests that the claimed impact on the employability of participants needs to be closely examined.

The Foundation: Federal/State Vocational Rehabilitation

The federal/state vocational rehabilitation program is the cornerstone of the vocational rehabilitation system.[1] Founded more than a half century ago, it experienced rapid growth during the last decade. In fiscal 1965 under the basic grant program,

441,000 cases were served and 135,000 successfully rehabilitated (Fig. 2-1). In the next decade, the annual case load grew to 1,143,000, including 306,000 rehabilitations, and outlays increased more than fivefold to $869 million. The federal government contributed the lion's share in its partnership with the state, accounting for 77 percent of funds in fiscal 1975 compared to 62 percent a decade earlier. Adding reimbursed services for public assistance and disability insurance beneficiaries, the total price tag for federal/state vocational rehabilitation activities in fiscal 1975 was over $1 billion. Despite this rapid growth, however, there has been a basic continuity in administrative approach, client selection, and services.

Administrative Approach. Vocational rehabilitation agencies operate in each state, with a number of local offices. The disabled are referred from a variety of sources and are usually assigned immediately to an individual counselor who collects basic data to determine eligibility. Those who have verified disabilities that are a substantial handicap to employment and who can be expected to improve with help are eligible. Those not accepted may be referred elsewhere and they may appeal the decision. When it is uncertain whether the applicant can be helped, he or she may be accepted for evaluation of up to 18 months during which time nonvocational services are provided and assessments made. At or before the end of this period, the applicant is either added to the active case load or is dropped.

All those who are accepted join a counselor in developing a rehabilitation program outlining goals and needed services. The counselor then arranges for the delivery of services that can include counseling, physical restoration, training, education, maintenance, work adjustment, placement, help in establishing a small business, social services, or other aid. In theory, the resources for any single client are unlimited, depending solely on individual needs. The counselor and other rehabilitation agency personnel may deliver the designated services, or purchase them from private or public sources. Participants who find

Figure 2-1
FEDERAL/STATE VOCATIONAL REHABILITATION OPERATIONS, FISCAL 1960-1975

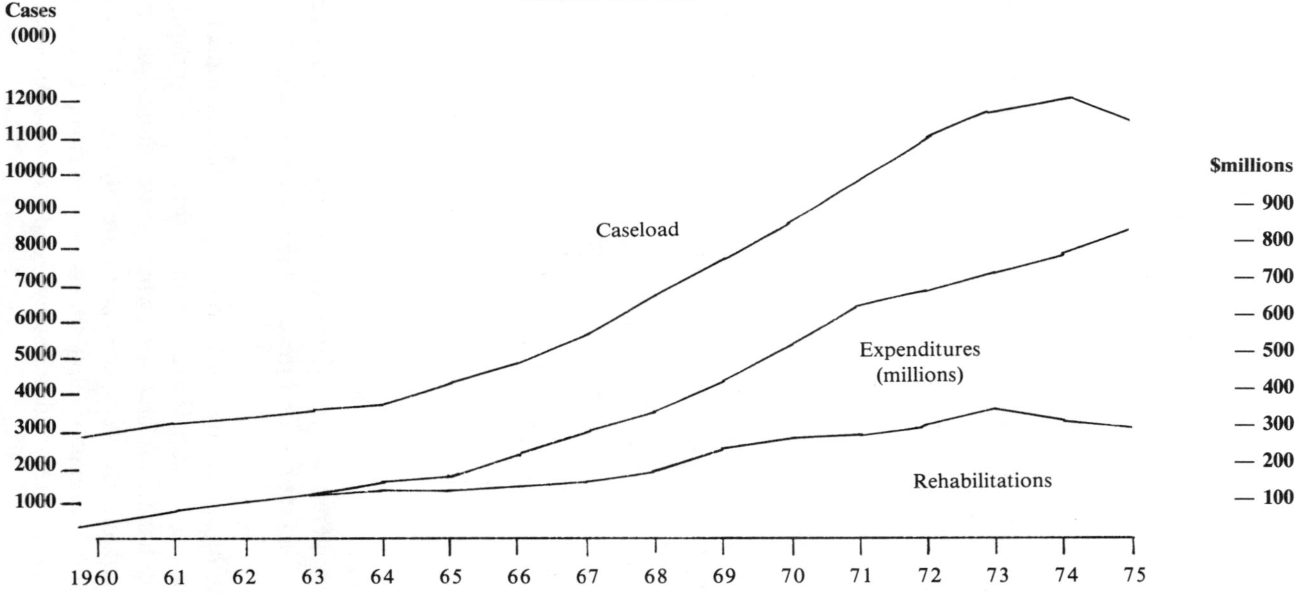

Source: U.S., Department of Health, Education and Welfare, Rehabilitation Services Administration, "Information Memorandum RSA-IM-76-29" (October 1975). (Mimeographed); U.S., Department of Health, Education and Welfare, Rehabilitation Services Administration, *State Vocational Rehabilitation Agency Program Data, Fiscal 1971*; Sar A. Levitan and Garth Mangum, *Federal Training and Work Programs in the Sixties* (Ann Arbor, Mich.: Institute of Industrial and Labor Relations, 1969), p. 283.

a competitive job and hold it for two months, homemakers with improved functional capacity, persons moving into permanent employment in sheltered workshops, unpaid family workers, and the self-employed are all counted as "rehabilitated." Those who drop out or complete their service program without employment are counted as nonrehabilitants.

Client Selection. The screening process seems to select the potentially most successful candidates either because of their own perseverance or the predilections of vocational rehabilitation counselors. In FY 1967 social security disability insurance recipients, who by definition are very severely disabled, represented 26 percent of the nonrehabilitated compared with 13 percent of those who were rehabilitated. Their 16 percent share of cases closed in that year was substantially less than their 24 percent share of rejected referrals and applicants. Persons 45 and over represented 28 percent of all active cases closed but 35 percent of those not accepted for services.[2] Applicant rejection rates averaged a third lower for the high success potential groups compared to those with more limited prospects.[3]

In surveys, counselors indicate that they try to mix their caseloads, balancing some who will require relatively extensive treatment with individuals needing lesser assistance. In FY 1973, 15 percent of unaccepted cases were persons with handicaps too severe to be served, while 14 percent were those whose problems were judged not severe enough. But among the remainder, some reasons cited for rejection, such as the client's failure to cooperate or refusal of services, may have hidden the counselor bias that resulted in acceptance of those with higher potential.

Creaming is relative, however, and if the vocational rehabilitation program tends to select the disabled with somewhat less serious handicaps and somewhat greater commitment to improvement and recovery, the clients are still seriously disadvantaged. Two percent of rehabilitants are blind in both eyes, an equal proportion are blind in one eye, and the same percentage are deaf. A tenth have lower body impairments and an equal proportion are psychotic or psychoneurotic; One in eight is mentally retarded; other categories such as dental problems, hernias, hay fever, asthma, and mild hearing impairments other than deafness may be less severe on the average but these account for less than a tenth of rehabilitants.[4]

Participants are also socioeconomically handicapped. Only a third of rehabilitants in fiscal 1973 were in the prime working years (age 25 to 44), with more than two-fifths age 24 years or less; nearly a fourth were nonwhites; only two of five had completed high school, and more than a third had less than nine years of schooling. At referral, 17 percent were working and a similar percentage listed earnings as their primary source of support. Half relied on family and friends, the remainder on public aid. Some of these clients may have been experiencing only transitional physical or employment problems, and overall they may not have been as bad off as nonrehabilitants, the nonaccepted and the seriously disabled not applying for aid; yet they were clearly a group with serious problems.

Services. The vocational rehabilitation program offers substantial assistance to overcome these difficulties. Individualized treatment begins with the vocational rehabilitation counselor. In FY 1975, outlays for counseling and placement averaged $283 per client served. This included the costs of developing individual plans, arranging services, troubleshooting, and recordkeeping as well as job referral and guidance. The adequacy of these services is difficult to judge. According to one comprehensive survey, three-tenths of successful rehabilitants and nearly half of nonrehabilitants were dissatisfied with their rehabilitation plans or claimed that none had been prepared; less than half remembered receiving any counseling.[5] The most recent study of vocational rehabilitation counselor activities in Florida and West Virginia found that they spent less than 15 percent of their time in actual counseling; 45 percent was allocated to referrals, eligibility determination, planning and placement, and the rest to paper work or other activities.[6] This rough breakdown has been found in other studies. Placement is not given a major priority in most vocational rehabilitation offices. Only one in five successful rehabilitants in a large follow-up sample claimed they got any help from vocational rehabilitation counselors in finding a job, with one in seven securing their first job after service as a result of this assistance.[7]

While some rehabilitants have claimed that more guidance, counseling and placement services are needed,[8] there is no doubt that a broad range of services are available and frequently provided. Most participants receive diagnostic and evaluation services, which may mean a medical check-up or vocational tests in a sheltered workshop. The most common services are physical or mental restoration and training. Two of five FY 1973 rehabilitants had received restoration services. In FY 1975, 12 percent of all clients served were provided surgery and treatment, 9 percent prosthetic and orthopedic appliances, 5 percent hospital or convalescent care, and 1 percent other restoration.[9]

Roughly half of FY 1973 rehabilitants had received some training. Personal adjustment training (essentially work experience and instruction in self-care) was most prevalent, and together with college and vocational school offerings, accounted for roughly half of all trainees. The value of training is uncertain. Only a fifth of a sample of rehabilitants felt that training helped them directly in getting a job or that they used training very much in their current job.

Clients may also receive services from other agencies without the costs showing up in federal/state vocational rehabilitation accounts. A recent survey found that 23 percent of rehabilitants had been aided during or soon after participation by a welfare agency, 4 percent by the Veterans Administration, a fifth by private or public employment agencies, and an equal percentage by social security agencies. The proportions were even higher among nonrehabilitants.[10] A fuller accounting might include the costs of equal opportunity enforcement, of jobs created under special employment arrangements, of placements into public employment programs, and perhaps even some of the costs of job creation for the disabled within the vocational rehabilitation establishment.

With a personalized approach, thère is a very wide range in treatment levels. For all rehabilitants, the average time from acceptance to closure was 16.4 months in fiscal 1973, with a median of 11.6. More than a fifth had been on the rolls for two years or more, while a third were on 6 months or less. The vocational rehabilitation program spent an average of $821 to purchase outside services for those who were rehabilitated in fiscal 1973. Yet the outlay was over $3,000 for 5 percent of rehabilitants, while a tenth were provided with inside services and another 25 percent received less than $100 worth of purchased assistance. A fourth of rehabilitants thus received about two-thirds of the individual services purchased by the program.[11]

In fiscal 1975 outlays for the basic federal/state program amounted to $869 million. Reimbursed services for SSI and DI recipients accounted for another $48 and $77 million respectively, while innovation and experimentation expenditures added another $24 million. Of the total, roughly a fifth went for training and an eighth for physical and mental restoration. Counseling and placement accounted for a third, or combined with diagnostic and evaluation services, for about two-fifths.[12]

Evolutionary Changes. Between 1968, when Congress last overhauled the vocational rehabilitation program, and 1975, average expenditures per rehabilitant rose from $1,816 to $2,839, or by 7 percent adjusting for changes in the cost of living. In fiscal 1968, 35.6 percent of funds went for counseling, placement, and administration—the expenses of the vocational rehabilitation establishment. By fiscal 1975, this proportion had risen to 40.2 percent. Meanwhile, restoration and training expenditures dropped from 37.2 to 33.4 percent of outlays. This probably reflected a shift from more costly restoration services, although the data are not conclusive. The proportion of clients receiving surgery or treatment, which is relatively expensive, dropped from 12.0 to 11.5 percent between 1971 and 1975, and the proportion with hospital or convalescent care dropped from 6.2 to 5.2 percent.[13]

There has been an increased reliance on sheltered workshops. In fiscal 1965, 46,800 or a tenth of all clients were treated there, with payments to workshops representing a fourth of total expenditures. By 1975, the 223,700 vocational rehabilitation participants treated in workshops accounted for a sixth of the total, and payments represented three-tenths of all expenditures. The proportion of rehabilitants placed into permanent employment in sheltered workshops rose from 3.2 percent in FY 1968 to 3.8 percent in FY 1974.

In recent years, there have been some important changes in the characteristics of participants. The mentally ill were 19.6 percent of rehabilitants in fiscal 1968 but 31.4 percent in fiscal 1974; the retarded increased from 10.7 to 12.6 percent. Other disability categories fell commensurately. For instance, amputees and persons with orthopedic handicaps declined from 24.2 to 19.5 percent of all rehabilitants. Reflecting the expansion of income support, the proportion on public assistance rose from 11 to 19 percent over the six years while the proportion whose primary source of support was earnings fell from 20 to 16 percent.[14]

The Vocational Rehabilitation Act of 1973 mandated increasing services to the more severely handicapped. In FY 1974, 114,000 or 32 percent of all rehabilitants were severely disabled according to the initial definitions developed by the Rehabilitation Services Administration. The number of nonseverely disabled rehabilitants dropped in FY 1975 but the severely disabled rose to 116,000 or 36 percent.[15] In the first quarter of fiscal 1976, 38 percent of rehabilitants were severely disabled as were 41 percent of the cases newly accepted for services.[16]

Slack labor markets in the 1970s, an expanding case load, and a more disadvantaged clientele adversely affected placement rates. In 1963, 80 percent of closed cases were rehabilitated successfully. In 1972, when the national unemployment rate was roughly the same, the success rate had declined to 75 percent. With the severe middecade recession, rehabilitations fell to 70 percent of closures in fiscal 1975 as the absolute number of rehabilitations dropped for the first time in two decades. In the first quarter of fiscal 1976, the rehabilitation rate was only 62 percent.

The shift to a more severely disabled clientele after the 1973 legislation was a minor factor in the mid-1970s performance slump. In the first quarter of FY 1976, the success rate of the severely disabled was 59 percent compared to 65 percent for those with less severe problems. This difference, multiplied by the several percentage point increase in the proportion of clients severely disabled, could have reduced average success probabilities very little. Over the longer run, however, changes in clientele can be important. The rehabilitation rate in fiscal 1970 of participants with mental illness or mental retardation was 72 percent compared with 81 percent for all other participants. The increase between 1968 and 1974 in the proportion of clients with a mental affliction could have contributed to a 1 percentage point decline in rehabilitation rates.

Performance.   Is this complex rehabilitation system effective in achieving its goals of restoring productivity, increasing earnings, and reducing dependency on public transfers? Rehabilitants in 1973 had earned an average of only $14 weekly at referral. Four-fifths had no earnings, while the remainder who worked averaged $72. At closure, 85 percent were receiving wages, averaging $76 weekly for all rehabilitants and $90 for those with earnings. At referral, 17 percent of rehabilitants were receiving public assistance; upon closure, only 8 percent.[17]

While these average gains are substantial, many rehabilitants remain below minimal levels of self-support. In FY 1973, 15 percent of rehabilitants had no earnings, 10 percent earned less than $40 weekly, and 28 percent between $40 and $80. In other words, less than half of supposedly successful rehabilitants found jobs where they earned the equivalent of the full-time minimum wage.

Earnings gains cannot be ascribed to services alone. Clients are selected on the basis of their employment problems, and in any group of unemployed the chances of improvement outweigh the possibilities of deterioration. In other words, the earnings at entry may reflect temporary employment difficulties. According to one sample of rehabilitants, wages and salaries in the three months prior to entry were 34 percent above those projected from the referral week status; earnings in the previous year were 53 percent higher.[18] A national survey of FY 1971 closures found that annual earnings in the calendar year before entry were $1,525 for rehabilitants, double the earnings that would have been realized from 52 weeks of employment at the weekly rate on referral.[19]

Earnings at referral are an accurate indication of future prospects only for those who have in the recent past suffered a deterioration in their physical or mental condition that is likely to be permanent. If the disabilities are of longer standing, or if previous earnings are correlated with future success changes, then a longer base period is more appropriate. The choice makes a significant difference. For instance, the national survey of 1971 rehabilitants found annual earnings rose from $1,525 in the prereferral year to $2,225 in 1971, or by 46 percent. Projections from the program data collected at entry and closure implied a gain from $750 to $3,353, or more than a fourfold increase.

Not counted in these earnings data are the benefits that accrue to the one in seven rehabilitants who is a homemaker. The economic value of a homemaker's service is difficult to determine. One reasonable valuation of a year's work is around $5,000.[20] On the other hand, among the two-fifths of disabled women who reported needing household help in 1966, three-fourths got it free and the other fourth paid out a median of $8 per week or $416 per year. If vocational rehabilitation services turned those performing no duties into proficient homemakers with a $5,000 output, then this would be a major achievement. If the result were merely to alleviate the need for purchasing outside services, the results would be less substantial. According to a 1973 survey of rehabilitants, the percentage reporting currently doing more housework was only 11 percent, barely higher than the 9 percent reporting doing less. Improvements were only slightly higher for persons who had initially been homemakers than for nonhomemakers.[21]

The duration of program impacts is another crucial issue. A person is counted as rehabilitated if he or she is gainfully employed for two months or demonstrates improved homemaking capability. But how long will employment or other improvements continue? A Minnesota follow-up of cases closed to employment between 1964 and 1967 showed that nearly four of five were still working in 1968. A 1970 Wisconsin survey of fiscal 1966–1968 rehabilitants found 68 percent employed, while a one-year-after review of fiscal 1968 and 1969 rehabilitants determined that between 65 and 73 percent were still employed. A 1974 Michigan study of fiscal 1970 closures and a separate 1973 sample in California and Pennsylvania both found 57 percent were still working one to three years after rehabilitation.[22] Finally, two-thirds of rehabilitants placed into a remunerative position in FY 1970 were still working according to a 1972 General Accounting Office survey.[23]

Because the vocational rehabilitation system operates as a sorting mechanism, its clients are more likely to succeed than those not accepted. Similarly, rehabilitated clients are more advantaged than those who are not rehabilitated. The gains of rehabilitants are not the sole result of services, and comparisons with nonrehabilitants or persons not accepted exaggerate the impacts of services.

There is, for instance, a sizeable portion of the case load that receives only limited services not likely to have a significant impact on long-run employability. One must question whether assistance really "rehabilitated" the third of the successes receiving purchased services costing less than $100. While a wheelchair, a cane, or glasses might be extremely useful or essential, many of the clients could afford to purchase these lower price aids. Rehabilitants are in the best position to judge the impact of services. Only 45 percent of rehabilitants in one recent sample felt that they had successfully completed rehabilitation. Of those with negative assessments, one in three claimed they received no services, two-fifths did not feel they completed their plan, and one in ten completed but could not find a job. Of this same group, a fifth continued in the same job, 7 percent sought other means of rehabilitation, and a third stayed home or were unemployed.[24]

How many clients reported as rehabilitated merely moved through the system on paper or received only marginal attention? If only half are given intensive assistance and if the wage gains are realized by those who improve on their own because of less severe problems, then the effectiveness of services for those most in need may be very much less than the aggregate figures suggest.

With all these caveats, there is little doubt that the federal/state vocational rehabilitation program contributes to the significant improvements in employment and earnings realized by rehabilitants. Some are helped who might make it on their own, and others are given extensive aid despite their limited potential for competitive employment. But the average client has serious impediments to work that might not be overcome without some assistance. Rehabilitation methods and priorities may need some adjustment in light of a changing labor market and clientele, but on the average the program's approach still produces substantial results.

Without denying the value and overall effectiveness of the vocational rehabilitation program, it is still proper to suggest certain improvements. This cursory review does not provide the basis for detailed policy prescriptions, but it does raise some issues that should be further examined.

Vocational rehabilitation has enjoyed sustained growth. It is difficult, however, to assess the marginal impact of any single component of the expanding system. An increased proportion of outlays go for administration and a declining portion for services. As the trend continues toward serving the most seriously handicapped, placement will cease to be a valid and significant test of program effectiveness. More services will be needed by the more severely disabled, but output will become increasingly difficult to gauge, with a consequent loss of accountability. It is vital, then, to determine what is necessary and what is secondary. For example, doubts have been raised about the homemaking component. With no objective standard of successful rehabilitation as a homemaker, and no quantification of benefits, this can become a catch-all category. The limited evidence indicates that rehabilitation is having little impact on housework capabilities. Another questionable practice is the reimbursed rehabilitation of transfer recipients. The danger is that the treatment strategies that have been developed over the years will have diluted effectiveness, while paperwork will necessarily increase as the sources of funds multiply. Moreover, the failure to reduce welfare case loads appreciably will reflect on the overall federal/state program.

Perhaps the more important issue is the possibility of marginally declining effectiveness. The recession had a noticeable impact in 1974 and 1975, and if the 1973 experience is a reliable gauge, improved placement rates should be realized if there is a healthy recovery. Yet while secular changes in the labor market are reducing job opportunities for the severely disabled, the vocational rehabilitation program is giving this group increased emphasis, and placement rates are likely to suffer.

There is need, then, for a more careful examination of the vocational rehabilitation program. Control groups are vital to assess long-run impacts on clients. Attention must be given to the implications of serving the more disadvantaged in a slack labor market. Certain practices, such as the training of homemakers and the reimbursed rehabilitation of transfer recipients, should be subjected to careful scrutiny so that these do not undermine the primary objectives of the program. Finally, there is a need to cut down extraneous services and to improve efficiency. The value of vocational rehabilitation is undisputed, but because it serves those whose needs are most pressing, we should not relax the demand for the highest standards of performance.

The Underlying Issues

The Universe of Need

Vocational rehabilitation efforts seek to increase the employability of those who are limited by mental or physical handicaps, but not all disabled are feasible candidates. It is useful, therefore, to estimate the number of persons with serious needs who want and could benefit from rehabilitation services.

This is not a simple, straightforward procedure. By definition the disabled are limited in the kind or amount of work they can do. But some may have perfectly adequate earnings; others without earnings may be receiving income transfers; still others may have so little vocational potential that services could do little to enhance their employability. Any reasonable estimate of needs must screen out persons with less consequential difficulties as well as those with problems so severe that they can never be overcome and those who do not want help.

Estimates of need rest, of course, on a set of assumptions and value judgments. There are no hard and fast rules. Advocates of expanded services, who want to demonstrate unfilled needs, understandably utilize the assumptions that yield the largest estimates. Since vocational rehabilitation has enjoyed widespread support, and since most analysis has been done by "insiders," the prevailing estimates of need are probably on the high side.

Estimates of Needs

The five major universe of needs studies have yielded estimates ranging from 5.1 to 7.1 million for fiscal 1973.[25]

Based on a review of state plans, Harbridge House estimated that 3.43 percent of the population, or 5.1 million persons, were handicapped and could benefit from vocational rehabilitation services. At the opposite end of the spectrum, an estimate by Nagi which included all persons under 65 who had retired or left their last employment because of disability, were forced into part-time work, or could not perform housekeeping or school work, yielded the 7.1 million estimate. The three other needs studies by Ridge, Worrall and Schoon, and Berkowitz broke down the disabled population in need of vocational rehabilitation services into certain subgroups. Their more detailed calculations led to the following estimates: the disabled unemployed, 1.0 million (based on 1966 data, projected for 1973); disabled persons who were not actively seeking work but who would work if they had the opportunity, 1.4 million; the disabled underemployed, 1.0 million; disabled homemakers, 1.7 million. In sum, these estimates yield a total universe of need of 5.1 million. If persons with secondary work limitations (able to work regularly in the same job) were excluded on the assumption that their needs were not severe, the target population would be reduced to 3.5 million.

If vocational rehabilitation caseloads are compared to the estimated 3.5 to 5.1 million persons in need of services—as they have been by advocates of expanded aid—there would appear to be major service deficits. The vocational rehabilitation program served between 23 and 34 percent of the target population in fiscal 1973 depending on which estimate is used; it accepted somewhere between 10 and 14 percent and successfully rehabilitated between 7 and 10 percent.

Reducing Needs Definitionally

Yet under equally or even more reasonable assumptions, the estimated universe of need is reduced substantially, and the service deficit lowered correspondingly. First, the inclusion of disabled homemakers in the needs estimate should be questioned. Because there is no standard for determining who needs aid or what the benefits and costs may be, and because the considerations in serving homemakers are different from those in serving labor force participants, it might be more appropriate to consider two universes of need. If homemakers are excluded from the above estimate of needs, the number of disabled persons in need of employment-related services drops to 3.4 million, counting those with secondary work limitations, or 3.0 million excluding them. In order to compare this estimate of the population in need with the population served, the individuals trained in homemaking are subtracted from the total number of rehabilitants. If the figures are adjusted to exclude homemakers, the percentage of estimated universe in need who received employability services would rise to 30–34 percent.

The universe of need is further reduced if the estimates of unemployment are based on 1972 survey data. In that year, only 710,000 disabled were jobless, or 485,000 excluding those with secondary work limitations, compared to the estimated 979,000 and 680,000, respectively, projected for 1973 from 1966 data.

A third estimate cited in the universe of need studies—the figure of 1.4 million disabled in 1973 who were not in the labor force but wanted a job—might be challenged. While 12 percent of those not in the labor force because of illness or disability claimed they wanted a job now, many of those with disabilities apparently did not think their disability was the reason for not seeking work. There were only 619,000 persons in 1973 who claimed they wanted a job currently but were not looking because of either illness or disability, and some of these were merely ill rather than disabled. Furthermore, subjective responses to job desire questions are difficult to interpret. Many of the disabled may want a job but are unable to work because they are too incapacitated. Others may claim to want a job because it is socially acceptable, but really have little desire. The overwhelming majority of the disabled who quit working after onset did so in accord with doctor's orders or their own desires to quit and not because they believed jobs were unavailable. Assuming arbitrarily that half of the 619,000 are disabled, desire employment, and can feasibly work with assistance, the universe of need would be 310,000, including 60,000 persons with secondary work limitations.

Finally, the estimate of 1.0 million underemployed disabled workers is probably understated. The 1972 survey found that among the 6.7 million disabled who are employed, 18 percent earned under $50 weekly. This estimate of the underemployed would yield 1,179,000 persons in 1972, including 259,000 persons with secondary work limitations.

Using these alternative figures (and assuming they held true for 1973 when economic conditions improved), the universe of need would be 2.2 million, or 1.7 million excluding those with secondary work limitations.

The practice of comparing the total number of individuals served by the vocational rehabilitation program to *any* needs estimate is in itself misleading. Such a comparison exaggerates the service deficit in two ways. First, the vocational rehabilitation program is only one possible service deliverer. If there is a deficit, it may make sense to expand the vocational rehabilitation program, but the deficit must be calculated by considering all providers. The federal/state vocational rehabilitation program is only one of several public providers, and the number of services arranged by this group is exceeded by the number of services arranged by private sources. Second, the ratio of services to needs compares a flow with a stock — that is, persons served each year with all persons disabled and in need of services.

It is difficult to estimate the annual number of persons who become disabled and need services or who experience a deterioration in their condition that creates a service need. The Rehabilitation Services Administration has estimated that there were 801,000 new potential clients in 1972, rising to 867,000 by 1977. Another study based on state plans came up with a figure of 912,000 annually.[26]

The basis for these estimates is unclear, but they appear to be on the high side. The 1971 Survey of Recently Disabled Adults found that 1.7 million persons became disabled between

October 1969 and March 1971. On an annual basis, this amounted to 1.2 million, including 574,000 severely disabled; 245,000 occupationally disabled; and 339,000 persons with secondary work limitations. Yet in 1971, more than a fourth of these newly disabled were employed full-time, compared with half the total work force.[27] If the differential is used as an estimate of the extra need generated by disability, this results in only 280,000 persons added annually to the disabled with serious labor market problems.

Additional need increments are generated when those already disabled suffer physical or economic setbacks. Among the 2.3 million disabled persons employed full-time in 1966, 573,000 were either not in the labor force, unemployed, or employed part-time three years later. If half of these are arbitrarily and conservatively assumed to be in need of services, the number coming into need over three years is 286,000, of whom a third may be assumed to enter the universe of need in any particular year. Adding the newly disabled and those with deteriorating conditions would suggest an annual flow of around 400,000 into the universe of need.

Measured against this total, the state/federal vocational rehabilitation program alone is exceeding the annual need, and thus cutting into the stock of disabled. Certainly this is the case if all rehabilitation services from all private and public deliverers are counted.

These crude estimates suggest some important considerations in weighing the adequacy of resources. While prevailing universe of need estimates have indicated large service deficits, the adoption of different assumptions yields much lower need totals and raises a new set of policy considerations. Because the provision of services to the disabled is worthwhile on the average does not mean that it is worthwhile at the margin, or in other words, that expansion is warranted. The possibility that vocational rehabilitation services meet a substantial portion of need makes it critically important to look at the margin. Is there a declining rate of return? Are expanded efforts feasible in a slack labor market? Can the universe of need be reasonably extended to include the more difficult to serve?

The Return on the Vocational Rehabilitation Investment

Central to vocational rehabilitation and manpower programs for the disadvantaged is the notion that public investments in human capital can be profitable. Services raise productivity and future earnings, and the present value of this stream of benefits can be compared with program outlays to calculate a rate of return. A benefit-to-cost ratio of 1.0 means that the services pay for themselves through subsequent gains of recipients. A ratio of 1.2 means that the return on the investment is 20 percent, comparing favorably to the payoff sought in business investments.

A number of studies in the 1960s purported to demonstrate the effectiveness of manpower programs for the disadvantaged, most frequently yielding benefit-cost ratios between 1 and 4 under standard assumptions.[28] In the early 1970s, these studies were challenged on several counts. Some critics claimed that control groups were poorly structured and others pointed to evidence from longitudinal surveys which showed diminishing returns over time. Their criticisms not only undermined the belief that manpower programs had succeeded, but also led some to conclude that they had failed.

In contrast, benefit-cost analyses of vocational rehabilitation yielded payoff rates so high that few questioned the value of these efforts. The major studies followed a standard format. The earnings before entrance to the program were compared with earnings subsequent to completion of rehabilitation. Base period earnings could include those in the week prior to entry, those in the quarter before, or those in the preceding year. Because the client may have been recently disabled, with prior year's earnings not fully reflecting present limitations, most studies used the entry status as a base. These pre- and postgains were projected under various assumptions. Some studies assumed that earnings at closure would continue to rise in real terms with general productivity increases; other studies did not. The likelihood of future job loss was considered, based on some follow-ups of rehabilitants; the typical assumption was that 15 percent of rehabilitants would lose their jobs in the first year; and an additional 5 percent in the next four. (Surprisingly, the probabilities that certain handicaps would become more severe and affect future work were usually ignored.) Some studies attempted to estimate the benefits to homemakers, while others included welfare savings. On the cost side, there were a variety of adjustments: deducting income maintenance costs, adding services delivered by other agencies, adjusting for foregone earnings, and recognizing that some clients would return for more services.

Benefit-Cost Studies. Despite a range of assumptions within this general framework, the major studies of vocational rehabilitation yielded consistently high rates of return. A 1965 study by Ronald Conley utilizing national data for 1959 to 1963 found that at a 4 percent discount rate, benefits were 14 to 17 times costs. In a 1969 update, using 1958 to 1967 national program data, Conley found that the rates ranged from a high of 19 in 1958, using a 4 percent discount rate and estimating benefits based on earnings at entry, to a low of 3 percent in 1967, using full-year preentry earnings as a base and discounting at 8 percent. Based on 1966 national data, the Rehabilitation Service Administration estimated that each dollar spent on vocational rehabilitation returned $36 in benefits, including the projected value of improved homemaking.[29]

More recent studies displayed greater sophistication in their assumptions and techniques, but the results were equally sanguine. An analysis of 1970 national data for a number of different groups by Monroe Berkowitz yielded a few cases of returns below 1, under the most conservative assumptions, but the overwhelming majority of benefit-cost ratios exceeded 10.[30] A study by Collignon and Dodson estimated a 14:1 return in fiscal 1972.[31] Abt Associates computed that benefit-cost ratios for the program in fiscal 1970 were 7 and 10 under the most conservative assumptions.[32]

The Importance of Methodology. These benefit-cost estimates for vocational rehabilitation exceeded all but the highest estimates for manpower programs. However, the methodologies used differed significantly. Manpower program studies frequently compared enrollees to others with similar characteristics, while none of the major vocational rehabilitation studies included control groups. Manpower program studies also tended to use more conservative assumptions in projecting benefits. The differences can best be illustrated by applying both the manpower and vocational rehabilitation benefit-cost approaches to the same data. One of the most comprehensive, if not the most technically sophisticated, analyses of any training program was a tracking by U.S. Department of Labor analysts of the earnings records of 55,000 1964 MDTA enrollees from 1958 to 1962 and subsequently from 1965 to 1969, using social security records.[33] A control group was selected from other records and matched according to age, race, sex, and prior earnings patterns. Since the social security records did not contain information on education, family status, or a number of other pertinent variables, the control group tended to be less disadvantaged than the trainees. Although this discrepancy may have resulted in an understatement of the impact of training, the basic data can be used to demonstrate the implications of alternative methodologies.

In comparing the absolute income gains of trainees and controls, the analysts found that training seemed to have had little impact. Between 1962 and 1965, the full calendar years before and after participation, enrollees increased earnings $58 more than controls. Thereafter, earnings of controls advanced more rapidly, so that the 1962 to 1969 gain for trainees was $61 less than that for the matched group. Even under the liberal assumption that the first year $58 differential in favor of trainees would continue for 5 years, the total gain at a 6.5 percent discount rate would amount to $257, compared with costs per enrollee of $1,665, thereby yielding a benefit-cost ratio of only 0.15.

Since the control group started with higher average earnings, similar gain rates would lead to widening differentials in favor of controls. Comparing rates of gain rather than absolute differentials, therefore, yields a somewhat more favorable picture. Between 1962 and 1965, the earnings of controls rose 75 percent while trainees enjoyed a 90 percent rise. If there had been no differential, trainees would have earned $174 less in 1965. Likewise, if trainees' earnings had grown at the 176 rate of controls rather than 196 percent rate achieved between 1962 and 1969, they would have been $227 less in the latter year. Assuming a 20-year future work life and a 6.5 percent discount rate, the benefit-cost ratio would be 2.1. Whether this ratio is more appropriate than the smaller one calculated above is debatable, but the difference suggests the range of assumptions usually applied in manpower benefit-cost studies.

The picture changes rather markedly when vocational rehabilitation benefit-cost methodologies are used. As noted, vocational rehabilitation studies focus on pre- and postchanges in the earnings of completers. If this approach is applied to the manpower training data, the programs take on the appearance of spectacular success. Between 1962 and 1965, the average earnings of completers rose $1,125. They then increased $710 in real terms by 1969, or roughly 7 percent annually. If discount and real growth rates of 6.5 percent are assumed, as well as a 20-year work life, the current value of the future gains would be $22,500. Divided by the $2,500 cost per completer, this would yield a benefit-cost ratio of 9.0 or more than 4 times as high as the more liberal ratio calculated using the control groups.

While the assumptions are simplistic, the exercise illustrates the implications of the differing approaches used in calculating benefit-cost ratios. Differences in assessment methodologies, rather than performance, may account for the much more positive judgments of vocational rehabilitation than of manpower programs.

Questions and Uncertainties. Base period earnings would indeed be predictive if the status of the disabled could not be expected to improve without the receipt of services. Among any group of handicapped persons with employment problems, however, some will recover, some will adjust, and some will get whatever assistance they need on their own. The extent of improvements will depend not just on services, but on the characteristics of the persons involved. For instance, the 1969 follow-up of persons disabled less than 10 years and not in the labor force in 1966 revealed that one in eight were employed in 1969. A fourth of those under age 45 found employment, with the proportion two-fifths among males in this age group. Over half of those with some college education improved their disability status or recovered between 1966 and 1969, twice the proportion among those with less than an eighth-grade education. More than half of all disabled persons working before onset of their disability were employed in 1966, compared with less than two-fifths of those not previously employed.

Prime age males with previous work experience and a high school education are overrepresented among persons receiving vocational rehabilitation relative to their proportion in the disabled universe. The types of persons served are thus likely to have a better chance of recovery and improved employment than others among the disabled. Rehabilitation services cannot be credited, therefore, with all the improvements realized by rehabilitants.

The long-run impacts of services cannot be determined just from future changes in the employment status of recipients. As the manpower training data suggest, there might be an initial improvement followed by a drop-off for trainees, compared with a steady increase for controls. According to a vocational rehabilitation follow-up study covering 1971 closures, the increase in earnings from the preentry to postclosure years was 48 percent for rehabilitants, −19 percent for nonrehabilitants, and −28 percent for persons not accepted. In the subsequent year, annual income for the "successes" rose only 8 percent compared with 23 percent for the other two groups, thereby closing the gap.[34]

Liberal projection techniques frequently inflate benefit-cost ratios of the vocational rehabilitation program. For instance, the financing of services from the DI trust fund is based on the notion that the savings resulting from possible benefit terminations will more than equal the costs of services. Through 1973, 13,000 recipients of reimbursed services had left the rolls. The value of cumulative expenditures was estimated to be $127 million, compared with $317 million in potential transfer savings. The benefit-cost ratio was, thus, a respectable 2.5 for service expenditures in the fiscal 1966 to 1973 period.[35] Based on such promising findings, the percentage of trust funds set aside for financing rehabilitation services was increased in fiscal 1973 and 1974. Yet in a deteriorating economy, there was a substantial decline in performance during the 1970s. Using standard assumptions, the ratio of annual savings to expenditures declined steadily from 3.8 in 1968 to 1.7 in 1973.[36] More critically, the assumptions used to estimate these returns were invalidated as performance declined. In FY 1974, 2,200 beneficiaries who were removed from disability insurance rolls reclaimed their eligibility; their numbers exceeded the total who had returned to social security rolls between FY 1966 and 1973.[37] More persons recidivated than terminated in fiscal 1974, and the number actively terminated declined from 12,991 the previous year to 11,796, suggesting negative marginal returns on the $56 million fiscal 1974 outlays. Earlier assumptions that those removed from the rolls would remain self-supporting were clearly invalidated.

An equally serious deficiency is the lack of real or simulated control groups to measure the impact of services. According to the law, clients chosen for reimbursed treatment should be those likely to leave benefit rolls with, but not without, aid. Rehabilitation agencies seek trust fund financing for recipients among their clients who are more likely to succeed. A GAO study examined 350 cases who were rehabilitated and who moved off social security disability rolls. In 51 percent of these cases, the individual had been scheduled for medical reexamination by the disability determination unit because of the possibility of recovery and regained earning capacity. Another 11 percent returned to work without receiving substantial rehabilitation agency services, and should not have been counted. Using the same methodology that yielded a 1.7 benefit-cost ratio for FY 1973, but excluding benefits from those not served or those possibly recovering on their own, the payoff would be reduced to 1.2.[38] If the subsequent national increase in recidivism rates had been factored into the calculations, the benefit-cost ratio would have been substantially less.

Lacking control groups, almost all vocational rehabilitation benefit-cost studies are seriously flawed. While they have grown increasingly sophisticated as researchers attempt to get around this shortcoming, the studies still overestimate the net impact of services. The return on the investment in the disabled may not be greater than that for helping other disadvantaged groups. If benefit-cost analysis is to be used to aid in policy decisions, then more realistic approaches are needed.

Client Priorities

The disabled range from functionally dependent quadraplegics to asthma sufferers. They include persons who have never worked, those with limited skills and education, and others who are afflicted with transitional problems as they adjust to their disabilities. The population also includes, however, some who are fully employed and drawing good salaries. In rationing scarce resources, a decision must be made whether to serve those with more serious physical and socioeconomic problems, or to concentrate on those closer to the margin of successful employment. Different services are required or are feasible for different groups of clients, and the chances of successful rehabilitation after such services vary.

Success Probabilities and Costs.   The first step in setting priorities is to determine differential costs and success probabilities. This information is relatively straightforward. The next step, estimating and comparing the relative benefits and costs, is less clear-cut. The conclusions require guesses about what would have happened to different clients in the absence of services and how long their employment gains will last. The final step is to factor in value judgments: how should efficiency considerations be weighed if they conflict with normative targets?

It is extremely difficult to analyze such questions. For instance, sheltered workshops concentrate on the most severely handicapped while the federal/state vocational rehabilitation program serves a mixed clientele. The institutional arrangements are completely different, the benefits and costs largely uncertain, and the normative issues conceptualized differently for each separate effort.

Problems of definition further complicate the effort to establish client priorities. To measure the relative effectiveness of services for the severely disabled, the selected group must be identified. The Rehabilitation Act of 1973 directed the Department of Health, Education and Welfare to develop a definition of the severely handicapped that would take into account the seriousness of mental or physical disabilities in terms of impairments to self-care, mobility, and self-direction as they affect employability, and also to consider disabilities in terms of the requirements for multiple and extended rehabilitation services. The tentative definition concentrated on disabling conditions. It included, for example, those with total blindness, loss of a limb due to orthopedic problems or amputation, psychosis, moderate and severe retardation, and heart disease. But while the chances of successful rehabilitation clearly vary with disabling conditions, they also vary with age, education, and other demographic factors. In FY 1970 the successs rates for orthopedically handicapped males in the federal/state program were: whites age 35–44, 9–11 years of education, 0.73; nonwhites age 35–44, 9–11 years of education, 0.69; whites under age 25, 9–11 years of education, 0.80; whites age 35–44, 12 or more years of education, 0.77.[39]

The costs of services vary significantly among different

client groups. Generally, high costs are associated with the treatment of those with greater success probabilities.[40] Multiple regression analysis of 1970 national data revealed that all else being equal, it cost $125 more to help 25- to 34-year-old rehabilitants than 45- to 54-year olds, and $131 less for high school dropouts than graduates.[41]

Allocation of Scarce Resources. Because higher costs are sometimes incurred in treating those with greater success probabilities, benefit-cost ratios are not always correlated with rehabilitation rates. In fact, one major study comparing earnings gains and costs for different groups concluded that if economic efficiency were to be taken as the criterion, it might be as desirable to focus on "the uneducated, the middle-aged, the severely disabled, the nonwhite, the unmarried and other low productivity groups as their more vocationally successful counterparts."[42] This study did not cross-classify education, age, race and handicaps in any detail, and more technically sophisticated regression analyses produced opposite conclusions. One study using a number of variables and analyzing 1969 data for the state of Florida showed that it was less desirable on efficiency grounds to help older unmarried, less educated, or severely disabled workers; nonwhites, however, were apparently a better investment than whites.[43] An even more detailed study using national FY 1970 data reached similar conclusions.[44] Another analysis, which compared all participants with the most severely handicapped as defined by the Department of Health, Education and Welfare, found that at a 7-percent discount rate, benefits were 16 times the costs for the program as a whole but only 9 times as great for the severely handicapped.

The consensus reached by these benefit/cost regression analyses does not, however, prove that it is more effective to serve the less disadvantaged. First, the calculation of the marginal impact of a number of different variables on payoff rates is a useful exercise, but the more policy relevant approach may be the simpler one of proceeding from cruder classifications. If most of the aged, for instance, have limited education and multiple impediments, the issue is not whether age may have one effect and limited education another, but whether these individuals on the average will benefit from services.

More critically, the assumptions used in estimating initial benefits and projecting them into the future are not neutral. Lower discount rates or more liberal assumptions about the continuance of gains will yield comparatively higher ratios for younger participants, and for those experiencing a greater improvement at a higher cost.

Without control groups, or at least some refinement of benefit measurements and projection assumptions, benefit-cost analysis is of little help in determining the relative efficiency of serving different clienteles. It is a useful exercise, illustrating that performance should not be judged by rehabilitation rates alone, but it provides no clear answers.

The assessment of the needs and potential of different client groups is not an exact science, and attempts to dictate priorities by detailed national guidelines are bound to be frustrated by diverse local approaches. Yet, on the average, reduced or increased pressure on placement or the provision or retrenchment in funds for services will influence behavior at the local level. The recent increases in the proportions of vocational rehabilitation clients found to be most severely handicapped may, in part, be a numbers game, but over time the composition of clients is changing and will continue to do so.

Whatever the cost-effectiveness of rehabilitating the more severely disabled, increased emphasis on serving them may mean that the average placement rate for the federal/state program as a whole will fall. A declining rehabilitation rate is not in itself an argument against serving the more severely disabled since higher rehabilitation rates are not necessarily indicative of higher benefit-cost payoffs. There is, in fact, no rigorous basis for choosing between alternative clienteles. There are some reasonable grounds for questioning the current emphasis on the needs of the severely disabled, however.

First, structural and cyclical changes in the labor market have pushed the disabled farther from the hiring door, so that the locus of most effective activity probably has to move forward along the labor queue. Second, the most severely disabled are most likely to have transfer income alleviating need while complicating rehabilitation efforts. Third, a decline in average future performance of vocational rehabilitation may adversely affect congressional support, leading to cutbacks or slower growth. Fourth, the acceptance of a more disadvantged clientele will mean acquiescence to lower placement rates. The removal of the market test may have adverse effects, disguising inefficiencies, or increasing unnecessary services. For instance, the performance of the federal/state employment service deteriorated by most measures when it emphasized the hard-core unemployed in the 1960s. The vocational rehabilitation program apparently worked well in the last decade. But the economic recession compounded the difficulties of the efforts to serve a clientele with more serious medical and economic problems. There are risks in trying to redirect an effective institution toward new goals unless the benefits are clear-cut.

The Service Mix

There are severe constraints on the "carte-blanche" treatment for the disabled under the federal/state vocational rehabilitation program. Resources are inadequate to provide everyone in need the services that would make them fully employable. Scarce resources must, therefore, be rationed among alternative services, delivery institutions, and clients, with the aim of attaining a mix that will have the most favorable aggregate impact. Regrettably, little is known about the relative costs, impacts, and needs for different services.

Individual counselors make decisions based on problem assessments, knowledge of available resources, and some common sense judgments about the effectiveness of different services, but they may have certain biases or be unresponsive to changing conditions. They may also be maximizing performance within a framework that is ill-designed for current needs and conditions. The available evidence raises some questions about the aggregate mix that results from counselors' separate decisions.

Content and Variability of Services. Counselors are central to the vocational rehabilitation process under both the veterans and federal/state programs, but little is known about their various functions. Studies of counselors' activities and interviews of clients suggest that much time is spent in arranging services and processing paperwork rather than providing help and guidance.

States vary markedly in their emphasis on counseling under the federal/state program. Maine, Massachusetts, Vermont, Arizona, Hawaii, and Oregon averaged 15 rehabilitants for every counselor in FY 1975. In New Jersey, Kentucky, Mississippi, Tennessee, and South Carolina, the average case load per counselor was four times higher. The states with more counselors achieved only 109 rehabilitations per 10,000 participants compared to 273 in the states with less counseling input. Whether the difference in performance is due to economies of scale or some other factor is uncertain, but if economies of scale are the answer, one would have expected that the rapid expansion of activity over the last decade could have been accomplished without a commensurate growth in counselors. The number of rehabilitations per counselor man-year fell from 45 in FY 1965 to 41 in FY 1974 and then to 31 in FY 1975, reflecting the sharply curtailed placement rate in 1975. Between 1967 and 1975, counseling and placement costs grew from 27 to 33 percent of total outlays.[45] Until it is proven that the services offered do make a difference, existing data cast serious doubts about the wisdom of expanded counseling, suggesting that it may, in fact, be a candidate for retirement.

The emphasis on restoration services also varies markedly under the federal/state program. In the ten states, less than one-tenth of FY 1975 expenditures for individual services went to buy physical and mental restoration. In marked contrast, the proportion was over 40 percent in eight states. Six states spent over 50 percent of restoration funds for surgery or treatment compared to five others spending 25 percent or less.[46] Average costs also varied markedly. Without medical expertise and some knowledge of the relationships between treatments and employability, one finds it difficult to say what is the ideal commitment.

"Training" covers a broad range of activities. College education is the primary emphasis of vocational rehabilitation for veterans. The constraints are the high cost, the lengthy treatment period, and the potential for serving only the most advantaged segment of the disabled population. But the benefits may be a permanent, quantum employability leap (although better documentation is needed before accepting this judgment). Vocational training in technical school or institutional skill centers can help the less educated. The problem is in bridging the gap between training and work. On-the-job training may be one solution, but it has not been tried for the disabled on any significant scale in the last decade. While the fragmentary evidence available suggests that it has had mixed success, on-the-job training does have the advantage of providing "earning while learning" and a job at the end of training. The difficulty is in getting employers to participate and in making sure that the persons hired are getting positions that would otherwise not be offered to them. Personal and vocational adjustment training accounted for 29 percent of training expenditures under the federal/state vocational rehabilitation program in FY 1975, but the nature and the effectiveness of the training remain unclear. Usually offered in sheltered workshops, it may provide clients with benefits that are transferable to competitive employment or it may merely prepare clients for their workshop assignments.

Once again, there is wide variance in the financing of the different training activities. In six states, over half of training funds under the federal/state program were devoted to college or university education. In contrast, over half the funds in four other states were spent on personal and vocational adjustment. While less than 4 percent of funds nationwide went for on-the-job training, three states spent proportionately four times as much.[47]

Job-creation strategies range from sheltered work to public employment. Workshops provide opportunities for those who have limited options. If the aim is work experience that will lead to competitive employment, only a small minority of participants have achieved it. If the aim is to supplement income and provide constructive activity at less cost than income transfers and recreation programs, then workshops are generally succeeding.

The Proper Recipe

Services provided by the federal/state vocational rehabilitation program differ from state to state. It is not possible to judge which service mix is most appropriate for each situation or to discern the implications of particular state programs for the optimum overall service mix.

Policymakers can, however, try to pin down the relationships between certain approaches and changing background factors. Job creation makes sense in a slack labor market. To the extent the more severely handicapped are served, the need increases for sheltered workshop opportunities. If the needs of a more select clientele are emphasized, public sector transitional jobs would be desirable. Flexible supported work programs, now being tested for groups such as addicts and alcoholics, are another alternative. In a tight labor market, on-the-job training might receive greater play, perhaps in the form of a special national subsidy program for employers hiring the handicapped. This strategy would be most effective when combined with affirmative antidiscrimination efforts. To the extent that the creation of jobs lessens the need for counseling and restoration, such services can be reserved for those who cannot perform in available slots.

These observations stop far short of identifying an ideal service mix. In the absence of hard evidence, judgments must be based on intuitions about the nature of the problems and the promise of different approaches. The employment perspective begins by concentrating on labor markets and the vocational dimensions of rehabilitation; predictably, it leads to greater emphasis on job creation and development. There is evidence, however, that the majority of potential clients would support this view of program priorities. When all the 1972 disabled and previously disabled who had received services from any source were asked what services they currently wanted, 67 percent of those with needs wanted vocational assistance and only 20 percent desired physical therapy or special devices. Among the recovered still desiring services, less than one-tenth needed restoration, but four-fifths wanted vocational assistance.

The message is not simply that restoration is being overemphasized. Rather, current restoration and manpower efforts for the disabled will have a greater impact if more attention is paid to the jobs that may be eventually secured. This means more than merely gearing up manpower services for the disabled; it entails creating new jobs and initiating antidiscrimination efforts and other insititutional changes. The disabled who are at the end of the labor queue need special assistance in overcoming institutional barriers and reestablishing or establishing a lasting job connection. Training and other services must be linked with jobs, and where jobs are not available they must be forged. Subsidies and job-creation programs can be used as mechanisms to change institutions. In short, there must be a renewed commitment to self-supporting employment, the primary goal of vocational rehabilitation.

Macroeconomic Considerations

The health of the economy affects everyone, but the impacts are greatest for the disabled and other labor force groups least prepared for work and least desired by employers. From 1963 to 1969 employment grew a vigorous 15 percent, and the number of unemployed fell by 30 percent. In the subsequent six years, the growth in employment declined to 9 percent and unemployment rose by 177 percent. Jobs were not available for many skilled and educated workers, but they were even scarcer for the more disadvantaged: the aged, the deficiently educated, and the minorities.

Even in the 1960s, however, the favorable effects of tight labor markets did not outweigh the combined secular impacts of higher minimum wages, technological change, and increased credentials requirements that made the unskilled and inexperienced workers expendable. Despite the increased availability of jobs, the difference in employment rates between male college graduates and those with 9 to 11 years of schooling widened between 1962 and 1969, as did the difference between the rates for white and nonwhite males and between the rates for older and prime age workers. The lean years of the 1970s merely accelerated these trends, or at least eliminated the compensatory growth of jobs.

These economic and labor force developments are best explained by the labor queue theory. Workers can be ranked according to their employability, which is a combination of their productive capabilities as manifested in previous job experience, skill-training, and formal education, as well as their attractiveness to employers (whether based on objective standards or biases). Those at the end of the line are much more likely to be jobless, much more likely to drop out of the labor force, and much less likely to find well-paying jobs. Some persons with limited education and experience may achieve great success, and steady employment in the past is no guarantee against failure, but success probabilities are largely determined by demographic and work experience characteristics.

The level of aggregate demand determines how far back down the labor queue employers will reach to fill their needs. In a tight labor market, more skilled and desirable workers are not available and employers have to be less selective. Those at the end benefit disproportionately in good times, since they are the source of labor that must be tapped for expansion. When aggregate demand declines, however, the last hired become the first fired, losing out in the competition with more attractive workers.

Human resource investment programs aim to increase the productivity of those at the end of the line, thereby raising their success probabilities. Antidiscrimination efforts, job restructuring, and other measures are designed to alter employers' standards and practices where these are unrelated to productivity. The goal of employment programs is to create jobs that will produce benefits for the individual and society in the form of productive output and reduced transfers.

At the End of the Queue. The labor queue notion is a useful device for understanding the problems of the disabled, who are more likely than the nondisabled to be older, black, and limited in their education, characteristics that would prove to be obstacles to employment even without physical or mental impairments. Moreover, in each age, sex, race, and educational attainment cohort, disabled workers have lower earnings and lower labor force participation rates. Employers prefer nondisabled workers, even if disadvantaged, to the disabled. There is also a queuing within the disabled universe. The chances of being severely disabled are related to the types of disabling conditions, with mental illness and retardation clearly having the most negative consequences.

The substantial annual inflow and outflow from the disabled universe is also explained by the labor queue notion. The chances of becoming disabled are highest and the exit probabilities lowest for those with unsteady work experience, limited education, greater age, and more severe handicaps. The key to continued labor force participation is the ability to remain in the same job after the onset of the disabling condition and this is quite clearly affected by whether the employer is hiring or laying off workers, and whether he considers the disabled employee valuable to the firm.

The impacts of secular and cyclical changes are evidenced by the sharp increase between 1966 and 1972 in the proportion of disabled persons unable to work regularly or at all regardless of the severity of functional limitation. The decline in work was greatest for those with the most serious physical and mental problems. The older cohorts and persons with limited education were hardest hit. As economic conditions deteriorated in the mid-1970s, the employment status of the disabled unquestionably suffered even more. Between 1971 and the third quarter of 1975, the number of persons aged 16 to 59 outside the labor force because of ill health or disability rose from 2.4 to 2.9 million, while the number among these claiming to want a job also rose, from 425,000 to 537,000.

Implications of Slack Labor Markets. The continuing high unemployment in the mid-1970s has important implications for vocational rehabilitation efforts. First, the composition of the universe of need has changed. Added to those with obvious work impediments are many disabled who have less severe handicaps and who would be able to find jobs and work productively in normal times. For these individuals, medical treatments will be less critical, because it is labor market changes that have pushed them out of the work force.

Second, deteriorating economic conditions reduce the absolute and relative success probabilities of the disabled, disproportionately affecting the most severely handicapped and disadvantaged. The employer who is willing to hire the disabled will now have a greater selection and will undoubtedly choose those with less limiting handicaps. For example, the mentally retarded, who have a slim chance of finding work in the best of times, will be competing with the orthopedically handicapped, who under normal conditions would be employed and who are preferred by employers.

Third, the relative effectiveness of various service strategies is affected by labor market changes. In a booming economy, on-the-job training, job development, antidiscrimination action and direct placement can be used to generate jobs for the disabled. These approaches will have an obviously reduced payoff when unemployment rises. When there are job deficits, work experience and public employment programs make more sense.

By the same token, medical treatment that may be adequate to lift many above the employability threshold in a tight labor market may not be enough to assure success when this threshold rises in a recession.

Fourth, hard times will force many who would otherwise be employed onto disability and relief rolls. Once the attachment to the labor force is broken, and the individual gets into the welfare system, complications arise in getting the person back into the job market. A worker who earns a livelihood may disdain dependency and view welfare as a complex and forbidding system. But once forced to depend on transfers, that individual may experience a change in values; fearing a loss of welfare benefits, he may come to regard work as the less desirable alternative.

Fifth, a slack labor market probably reduces the benefit-cost ratio of rehabilitation services while altering the relative payoff in serving different clienteles. Where the average client has a slim chance of employment without services, a slack labor market can reduce his success probabilities very little. But the success rate after services, which is normally high, can fall precipitously as placement becomes more difficult. The net payoff therefore declines.

These are probable, not proven, impacts of the 1970s economic slump. Data on the disabled and on vocational rehabilitation programs are too limited, and their interpretation is too uncertain, to establish a causal relationship with any certainty. Nevertheless, the available statistics on closure and recidivism in the rehabilitation program suggest that the rise in unemployment nationwide has had a marked effect. The ratio of successful to unsuccessful closures under the federal/state program declined from 3.40 for 1964 through 1968 to 3.07 during the subsequent four years.[48] It then dropped precipitously to 2.75 in 1974 and 2.28 in 1975. The recidivism rate of rehabilitants who had previously terminated from disability insurance rolls has ballooned; such a dramatic decline in job retention probably affects all previous rehabilitants.

Policy adaptations would seem to be appropriate what with the evidence supporting the theoretical probability that the disabled are seriously affected by labor market changes. Employment and training programs for the disadvantaged offer examples of possible changes. Public employment and work support efforts were expanded in response to the growing job deficit in the 1970s. In 1975, outlays for these efforts carried a $3 billion price tag, amounting to a fivefold increase in four years. Meanwhile outlays for training and placement declined (after adjusting for cost-of-living changes). Job creation increased from one-fifth of manpower outlays in fiscal 1971 to almost one-half in fiscal 1975 as total outlays doubled. There was also a noticeable shift to a less disadvantaged and better educated clientele.

In contrast, vocational rehabilitation policies were slow to adjust to changing conditions. While the recession probably doubled the number of nonworking disabled persons between the late 1960s and mid-1970s, federal/state vocational rehabilitation expenditures rose by less than two-fifths between 1971 and 1975. There was no major shift from training or medical services to public employment. The average number of clients in certified sheltered workshops rose by 50,000 in the early 1970s but expansion stopped in the face of the severe recession at mid-decade.

If macroeconomic developments have had the postulated effects on the disabled, then vocational rehabilitation policies should be brought more in line with general manpower policies. Such a revision would involve a deemphasis of service strategies designed to increase employability and a greater commitment to job creation and work experience efforts. It would also elevate the less disabled to a position of higher priority than the severely disabled. While there are no easy answers and no certainties, economic conditions must be given much greater consideration in the formulation of vocational rehabilitation policies.

Workfare and Welfare

Social insurance and welfare benefits are a major source of support for those with curtailed earnings. In 1971, half of all disabled household units received public support; social security aided nearly a fourth. One in seven received welfare benefits and one in ten veterans compensation. Social insurance benefits averaged $2,100 anually per recipient unit and public assistance, $1,500. Together they accounted for one-eighth of the aggregate income of households with a disabled adult, and almost a fourth for those with a severely disabled adult.[49] Since household survey data tend to substantially undercount transfer payments, and since the dollar totals do not include in-kind aid such as subsidized medical care, housing, food stamps, social services, and other assistance, the importance of government assistance is understated.

Growth of Income Support. Income support programs have been growing rapidly, and the disabled have become more and more dependent upon public support. The reported recipients of DI benefits and of public assistance for the blind and totally disabled increased by two-thirds between 1966 and 1972, while expenditures more than tripled. In the next three years, the combined case load rose by another two-fifths, or by a greater absolute number than between 1966 and 1972.

The DI total includes wives and dependent children. But the number of disabled workers alone rose from 1.1 million in December 1966 to 1.8 million in December 1972 and 2.5 million three years later. If the number of severely and occupationally disabled remained roughly constant between 1972 and 1975 as it did during the previous six years, this would mean that the percentage receiving benefits more than doubled. The growth rate of DI is also accelerating, with 0.6 million acceptances in 1966, 1.0 million in 1972, and 1.3 million in 1975.

Several factors contributed to this rapid growth. Legislative changes opened the doors to new claimants. Under the DI program, the definition of disability was changed in 1965 to include all incapacities expected to last a year or longer. Prior to this time, only individuals whose disabilities were of "long-continued and indefinite duration" were eligible for DI benefits.

In 1965 and in 1967, restrictions were eased for the younger blind, widows, and recipients of workers' compensation benefits. In 1972, the waiting period was reduced from six to five months. The black lung program was initiated in 1969 and significantly liberalized in 1972. In 1974 Aid to the Blind, Aid to the Totally and Permanently Disabled, and Old Age Assistance were replaced by the Supplemental Security Income (SSI) program, which introduced federal definitions of disability and encouraged states to expand benefits by footing more of the bill.

Another likely growth factor was the "greening" of the welfare and social insurance system, partially the result of court decisions and partially the result of changing attitudes in the welfare establishment. A major 1960 court decision held that disability determination under disability insurance required consideration not only of what the individual could do, but also of available employment opportunities. Where decisions had been made before on medical analysis of functional capabilities, the court held that the theoretical ability to engage in substantial gainful activity was not enough if no reasonable employment opportunities were available. To reestablish the priority of medical factors in disability determination, Congress changed the law in 1967, defining substantial gainful work to include any job existing in the national economy, whether or not job vacancies were available locally. Yet the door could not be closed.

In 1967, 70 percent of 466,000 cases requiring determination of disability were allowed. When the number of determinations rose to 852,000 by 1973, including more marginal cases, the preliminary approval rate fell to 63 percent, but increased reversals and court decisions held the final acceptance ratio nearly stable. Furthermore, roughly 75 percent of determinations in 1975 were made on the basis of age, education, and work experience, compared with only 10 percent in 1963. Medical factors are considered necessary but the other conditions have become increasingly crucial over time.[50]

The improvement in benefits was undoubtedly a major cause of growth. Between 1966 and 1975 the average benefit for the disabled worker more than doubled from $98 to $216, exceeding the rise in prices by a third, and the increase in real hourly earnings by a fourth. The addition of food stamps, subsidized housing, and Medicaid and Medicare benefits contributed to the dramatic improvement in the total benefit package.

Economic developments were also of central importance. DI is directed to those who cannot achieve substantial gainful employment, while public assistance is distributed on the basis of need and rather strict proof of physical limitations. When disabled persons were forced out of work by rising unemployment, they qualified for aid and in many cases had no other recourse.

Transfers as Work Disincentives. Yet the expansion of income support might also be the cause rather than the effect of reduced employment if the disabled reacted to more attractive benefits or expanded eligibility by shunning work. To the extent that this is the case, the changing employment patterns might reflect a pull rather than push out of the labor market, and therefore might not be indicative of reduced employment opportunities for those willing and capable of work.

A substantial difference exists between the work propensities of income transfer recipients and nonrecipients. A third of severely disabled males without DI benefits were working in 1972, four times the percentage among beneficiaries; 11 percent of unaided females with severe handicaps had jobs compared to 4 percent of recipients. The question, however, is whether DI merely aided those unable to work, as opposed to encouraging marginal workers to leave the labor market.

Regression analysis of 1966 data suggested that all else being equal, those with transfers worked less. Each $100 increase in annual transfers reduced the labor force participation rate by an estimated 0.6 percent for prime age white males and 1.1 percent for white males, aged 55 to 64. For blacks, the percentages were higher. An increase in real benefits of 33 percent, e.g., from $1,500 to $2,000 (roughly comparable to that occurring between 1966 and 1975), would reduce the labor force participation rate by 3.0 percent for disabled prime age white males and 5.5 percent for prime age blacks.

Other calculations using 1966 data found that for each increase of 10 percent in the ratio of benefits to average monthly wage in the last employment, the chances of application rose 2.4 percent.[51] If this were the case, the 25-percent increase in benefits relative to wages between 1966 and 1975 would have increased the likelihood of application by 6 percent. The increase in the incidence of application has far exceeded this amount.

Such calculations are inconclusive, but the data seem to support the commonsense judgment that the rise in disability rolls was not just the result of improved benefits and increased dependency propensities, but also the result of declining job opportunities.

Rehabilitation Instead of Relief. If employment opportunities were readily available for those receiving government transfers, it might be possible to help recipients prepare for jobs and to get them back to work. This has not proven easy, however.

Reimbursements for rehabilitation services from the disability insurance trust fund have been authorized since 1965 to get recipients back to work and off assistance. Up to 1 percent of disability payments could be used for this purpose initially, rising to 1.5 percent a decade later.

Through FY 1974, an estimated 300,000 beneficiaries received reimbursed services, and 75,000 in FY 1975. Reimbursements are also authorized from general revenues for rehabilitation services to SSI recipients, although only 3,600 were served in FY 1975. Under workers' compensation, rehabilitation may also be financed by private insurance or provided by referral to the public programs. According to scattered evidence, probably less than 5 percent of clients receive vocational rehabilitation.[52]

Are rehabilitation services a way to slow the growth of transfer program caseloads? The DI experience raises doubts.

Reimbursed services are reserved for beneficiaries who could be expected to return to competitive employment long enough so that savings from benefits will exceed rehabilitation costs. Earnings of $200 monthly are *prima facie* evidence of the ability to carry on substantial gainful employment, and those who reach this level of earnings face a possible cut-off in benefits. To mitigate the work disincentives, there is a year long trial work period before termination, and terminees who lose their jobs are automatically reeligible for benefits. Yet persons with earnings potential of only $2,400 annually and about the same level of benefits are not likely candidates for services. The system apparently favored the less disadvantaged as candidates for rehabilitation services.

Even among these selected clients, the success rates have been modest. Among the 52,000 trust fund financed cases served in FY 1973, 11,600 were closed successfully and 7,200 unsuccessfully; only 2,600 reimbursed rehabilitants were terminated from the rolls. Performance had deteriorated markedly as a larger proportion of recipients were drawn into rehabilitation efforts and as unemployment rose in the early 1970s. The cost per rehabilitant grew from $2,200 in FY 1969 to $3,400 in FY 1973, while the cost per terminee increased from $6,300 to $15,300. There was also substantial substitution of DI reimbursements for regular vocational rehabilitation expenditures. Total terminees declined as a proportion of disability beneficiaries, from 2.3 percent in FY 1970 to 1.6 percent in FY 1973, while service reimbursed recoverees fell from 0.17 to 0.11 percent. Clearly, there is little evidence that vocational rehabilitation can play a major role in countering the growth of disability insurance rolls.

In many ways, the 1970s explosion in disability benefits mirrored the earlier experience with welfare. In the late 1960s, Aid to Families with Dependent Children (AFDC) caseloads rose at an accelerated rate as a result of legislative changes, court decisions, liberalization of the welfare establishment, and most important, the improvements in welfare benefits relative to real wages. Public support fell as costs increased; welfare was blamed for causing family break-ups and for encouraging marginal workers to leave the labor force. Early efforts to halt growth through absolute ceilings, work incentives, and training services had little effect, so more rigorous measures were eventually adopted. Job referrals were made mandatory, benefits were allowed to erode, and more effective policing procedures were instituted to prevent abuse.

Disability programs have been cushioned by the public's greater acceptance of aid to those with obvious mental or physical handicaps. Nevertheless, recent case load increments have probably included persons with less serious problems who do not evoke as much sympathy, and there are signs that public and professional dissatisfaction with the system has grown. If costs continue to rise, policymakers are likely to adopt the same "get tough" stance assumed by their counterparts in the field of public welfare.

The Lessons. Experience with the welfare program suggests that for the majority of those individuals at the end of the labor queue who are affected by declining job opportunities and attracted by the increased minimum benefit, employment is not a realizable objective. The strategies that program administrators relied upon did not prove effective enough to offset the employment problems of the welfare recipients. It was found that job training did not ensure job placement, and that employers in the public sector were as wary of hiring recipients as employers in the private sector. The recession further reduced the chances of employment for the members of this group. The Work Incentive Program (WIN), which provided training and other services, may have been a worthwhile investment, but it did not remove a significant number of individuals from the welfare rolls and came under considerable criticism because of this failure. The lesson to be drawn from these efforts to place recipients in jobs is that the employment problems of those who turn to income support tend to be very severe and very difficult to treat.

A second lesson is that experimentation with benefit formulas is not likely to increase employment greatly. Many economists are critical of the use of cut-offs such as the substantial gainful employment cutoff of $200 monthly earnings under disability insurance. A recipient keeps everything up to this amount and still gets a DI check, but can lose it when earnings rise a dollar more (although this rarely occurs in practice). The answer would seem to be to introduce incentives as under WIN, where the recipient retains the first $30 of monthly earnings plus one-third of the remainder and work related expenses without offset. Yet after such incentives became effective in the late 1960s, work rates among welfare mothers did not increase noticeably. The introduction of incentives simply improved the status of recipients already working, and opened the doors to others who previously were not eligible because of their earnings. Changing the disability definition by allowing substantially higher earnings or permitting recipients to keep a portion of earnings would break down the notion of disability and would expand eligibility to the less seriously handicapped.

A third lesson is that growth will not necessarily continue exponentially. In the 1960s, welfare levels were raised and substantial in-kind benefits were added, improving the welfare package to poverty levels. Combined with a liberalization in eligibility standards, this change had the effect of making welfare a reasonable option for large segments of female-headed families. Within a few years, most of the families were on the welfare rolls. Near saturation of the eligible population and the stabilization of real benefits halted growth even in the face of a major recession. The boost in disability benefits under the SSI program likewise resulted in a spurt of recipients. As the recession levels off, as the universe of need is saturated, and as real benefits are raised less rapidly, the growth of disability beneficiaries will likely slow. Patience and compassion may be better policy than an aggressive effort to reform the disability system, to expand rehabilitation efforts or to get tough with applicants.

DIAGNOSIS AND PRESCRIPTION

Vocational Rehabilitation in the Context of Human Resource Development

Supported by a sympathetic public response and by claims of effectiveness in meeting the needs of the disabled, vocational rehabilitation has expanded at a rapid rate. Significantly, this growth has taken place independently of developments in other human resource programs. Policymakers and the general public have tended to view the disabled as a unique group, and as a result, vocational rehabilitation has established itself as a program distinct from other employment and training efforts.

There is some question, however, whether the employment problems of the disabled should be treated in isolation. An extensive overlap exists between the disabled and the socioeconomically disadvantaged. Many of the socioeconomically handicapped have complicating mental or physical problems, while a large proportion of those with mental or physical handicaps have limited education and limited work experience and skills. Both groups are positioned at the end of the labor queue and are alike in being affected disproportionately by structural and cyclical changes in the labor market.

Because the disabled and the disadvantaged share certain characteristics and must compete with one another for limited resources and scarce job opportunities, policymakers might be advised to adopt similar strategies in dealing with their problems. Decisions concerning the scale or mix of services, the selection of clients, and the question of income support should be made in a way that is consistent for both groups. Specifically, the vocational rehabilitation program might follow the lead of manpower programs by placing greater emphasis on labor market realities. The rehabilitation program still tends to view the problems of the disabled from a medical perspective; program objectives might be redirected to some extent from physical restoration to the improvement of client employability and the generation of jobs.

Finally, it would be useful to apply the performance standards of the manpower programs to vocational rehabilitation efforts. As this chapter has shown, benefit-cost analysis has played a significant role in judging the performance of both vocational rehabilitation and manpower programs. This type of analysis compares the cost of program services to the potential value of benefits to society and the individual participant in order to determine whether the investment has a positive rate of return. Most studies of vocational rehabilitation have found that benefits far exceed costs, with ratios substantially above those for general manpower programs. These findings have given momentum to the expansion of vocational rehabilitation, while the less favorable findings for manpower programs have led to reform and retrenchment. Yet the analyses that uphold the effectiveness of vocational rehabilitation are questionable and clearly less rigorous in their methodology than those used to test the performance of manpower programs. The rehabilitation studies have relied on comparisons of earnings immediately before and after rehabilitation, rather than comparisons of participants to matched samples of disabled nonparticipants over an extended period. Since many of the disabled recover or improve their employment status without services and since those with greater probability of improvement are selected for the program, before and after comparisons exaggerate the impact of rehabilitation efforts. Calculations with and without the use of control groups demonstrate that the differing methods used in assessing vocational rehabilitation and manpower programs have been responsible for the differing performance assessments. It is uncertain whether vocational rehabilitation pays off absolutely or relatively as a human capital investment. While chances are that it pays off on both counts, success is not as clear-cut as most existing studies would suggest. If policymakers are to have a more accurate understanding of the value of vocational rehabilitation, then the problems of creaming and control group adequacy must be faced squarely, and the program itself measured against the same kind of exacting standards as manpower efforts.

Other Issues

Cost-effectiveness is one consideration in evaluating the vocational rehabilitation program; the adequacy of services is another. Estimates of the universe of need are used to determine whether our present rehabilitation resources are sufficient to meet the needs of the disabled population. As the deficit between services and needs becomes larger, the justification for expansion becomes greater. Usually put forward by vocational rehabilitation advocates, estimates of need have been inflated by the inclusion of many who cannot feasibly be served, who are not interested in services, or who do not need them because of adequate employment on good chances of improvement. Some analysts have documented service deficits by confusing the total stock of disabled with the annual increment in need. Under conservative definitions, it can be demonstrated that the capacity of vocational rehabilitation programs exceeds the annual incremental needs. Although additional services and facilities may be required by worsening economic conditions, we currently appear to be much closer than many believe to meeting the needs of the disabled population in a comprehensive fashion.

Another important policy consideration concerns the impact of macroeconomic developments on the disabled. A precipitous decline has occurred in the number and proportion of the disabled who are employed, and many who would normally work despite their physical or mental handicaps cannot find jobs. The vocational rehabilitation system has been slow to adjust to the economic scenario of the 1970s and particularly slow to adapt its strategies to the lack of demand in the labor market. For example, a slack labor market undermines antidiscrimination, job development, placement, and on-the-job training efforts, but increases the need for public employment or sheltered work. It may also alter the relative payoffs in serving different clienteles. As the severely handicapped are moved farther and farther from the hiring door, the chances of eventual competitive placement are reduced. Economic conditions, then, would seem to call for the selection of a more moderately disabled clientele for the rehabilitation program. If those with less vocational potential are served, rehabilitation and placement rates will eventually fall, with ramifications for the rehabilitation system.

The optimal service mix remains an uncertainty. The marginal impact of specific treatments on different clients is unknown. Only a few general observations and a cataloging of questions are possible. Intake and assessment methods are more art than science, and they vary from counselor to counselor. The use of weighted formulas to influence client selection promises to complicate the situation. Counseling is a major part of all programs, but much of what goes by this name may involve paper shuffling and administration rather than the provision of services to the disabled clients. Training ranges from work experience to subsidized college education. Sheltered work fits in with public preferences, but it has yet to be proven that a job at subminimum wages is particularly therapeutic or rehabilitative. Institutional training of the disabled has uncertain results, while on-the-job training has been used sparingly. The returns to higher education for the disabled are probably significant, but not well-documented. Placement and job development have received very little emphasis in the federal/state vocational rehabilitation program or in sheltered workshops, and antidiscrimination efforts have not been pushed.

The increased incidence of income transfers raises other issues. DI, the black lung program, workers' compensation, and SSI have been expanding dramatically, suggesting the possibility that the disabled are being pulled rather than pushed from the work force. There have been some efforts to counter rising caseloads with rehabilitation services. These seemed to be effective at first, but as the economy slumped and the scale of activity rose, performance fell off precipitously. Experience with the rising AFDC rolls in the late 1960s and early 1970s suggests that neither training nor work incentives are likely to have much effect, and that expansion will level off once benefits stabilize at an acceptable real level and the eligible universe becomes saturated.

Policy Considerations

These issues are very complex, defying reduction into a straight forward agenda of policy prescription. Yet the preceding analysis suggests some policy considerations.

First, rapid growth in any institution involves some unnecessary "improvements" and unnecessary overhead. Vocational rehabilitation efforts have not escaped such developments. A rigorous assessment of rehabilitation institutions to ensure that waste is eliminated and that clients are served efficiently is overdue.

Second, nonvocational assistance such as counseling, evaluation, homemaking, and varied social services could probably be trimmed without affecting gainful employment goals. Nonvocational services may be justified and indeed necessary on their own grounds, but the impacts must be more clearly documented, especially in view of the fact that the persons prescribing needs are those delivering the services.

Third, jobs might be given greater emphasis. If the severely disabled are to be served, sheltered workshop opportunities can be increased by subsidizing employment and wages directly. Supported work and public employment programs could help the better qualified among the handicapped. Subsidized on-the-job training in the public sector might be initiated if the labor market tightens and if antidiscrimination efforts are mounted. Under all programs, employer outreach efforts are needed and placement services might be expanded.

Fourth, the emphasis on the more severely disabled should be reexamined. This is a complex issue, involving many value judgments. There are millions of persons with serious disabilities who can benefit from help. Policymakers should consider the possibility that the severely disabled would be better served with income support, given the limited employment potential of the most severely handicapped, and the considerable resource investment needed to prepare them for gainful employment. Scarce rehabilitation resources could be directed to individuals whose position in the labor market would be substantially improved.

Fifth, vocational rehabilitation should not be relied upon as the major strategy to counter rising welfare and DI caseloads. It may function well at the margin, but its potential is limited for those with handicaps so severe that they can qualify for transfer aid.

The purpose of this analysis was not to redirect policy, but to suggest different perspectives for decision makers. Labor market conditions must be a primary consideration in assessing efforts on behalf of the disabled. A greater understanding must exist of the overlap between disability and other obstacles that prevent workers from functioning effectively in the work force. The role of vocational rehabilitation in the galaxy of human resource development efforts must be recognized, policies coordinated, and experience cross-fertilized. There is no doubt about the importance of vocational rehabilitation in combatting the consequences of disability, but there is room for the improvement that will be realized by taking a new look at old problems.

NOTES

1. The account of the federal-state vocational rehabilitation program has been excerpted from the second chapter of the report *Jobs for the Disabled*. Since the present volume focuses on the federal-state program almost exclusively, the authors' discussion of sheltered workshops and

of the rehabilitation services provided by the Veterans Administration has been omitted. The complete version of the report is available in published form as Sar A. Levitan and Robert Taggart, *Jobs for the Disabled* (Baltimore, Md.: Johns Hopkins University Press, 1977).

2. U.S., Department of Health, Education, and Welfare, Rehabilitation Services Administration, "Length of Time Spent in Referral and Applicant Statuses by Selected Groups of Clients Whose Cases Were Closed During Fiscal 1967," *Statistical Note*, No. 6 (December 1967) (Mimeo).

3. U.S., Department of Health, Education, and Welfare, Rehabilitation Services Administration, "Major Disabling Conditions of Clients of State Vocational Rehabilitation Agencies Whose Cases Were Closed During Fiscal Year 1970," *Statistical Note*, No. 30 (June 1972) (Mimeo).

4. U.S., Department of Health, Education, and Welfare, Rehabilitation Services Administration, "Information Memorandum RSA-IM-75-28," November 1975 (Mimeo).

5. Abt Associates, *The Program Services and Support System of the Rehabilitation Services Administration* (Cambridge, Mass.: Abt Associates, Inc., 1976), pp. 213–215.

6. Abt Associates, p. 83.

7. Abt Associates, pp. 213–215.

8. See the follow-up of fiscal 1970 rehabilitants in U.S., General Accounting Office, *Effectiveness of Vocational Rehabilitation in Helping the Handicapped* (Washington, D.C.: U.S. Government Printing Office, 1973), p. 26.

9. U.S., Department of Health, Education, and Welfare, Rehabilitation Services Administration, *State Vocational Rehabilitation Agency Program Data, Fiscal Year 1975* (Washington, D.C.: U.S. Government Printing Office, 1976).

10. Abt Associates, p. 219.

11. U.S., Department of Health, Education, and Welfare, Rehabilitation Services Administration, "Information Memorandum RSA-IM-75-26," November 1974 (Mimeo).

12. U.S., Department of Health, Education, and Welfare, Rehabilitation Services Administration, *Agency Program Data, Fiscal Year 1975*.

13. U.S., Department of Health, Education, and Welfare, Rehabilitation Services Administration, *Agency Program Data*, Fiscal Years 1968, 1971, and 1975.

14. U.S., Department of Health, Education, and Welfare, Rehabilitation Services Administration, *Characteristics of Clients Rehabilitated in Fiscal Years 1968–1972* (Washington, D.C.: U.S. Government Print-

ing Office, 1974), and U.S., Department of Health, Education, and Welfare, Rehabilitation Services Administration, "Information Memorandum RSA-IM-75-28."

15. U.S., Department of Health, Education, and Welfare, Rehabilitation Services Administration, "Information Memorandum RSA-IM-76-22," August 1975 (Mimeo).

16. U.S., Department of Health, Education, and Welfare, Rehabilitation Services Administration, "Information Memorandum RSA-IM-76-63," March 1976 (Mimeo).

17. U.S., Department of Health, Education, and Welfare, Rehabilitation Services Administration, "Information Memorandum RSA-IM-75-28."

18. Abt Associates, p. 181.

19. Joseph Greenblum, "Evaluating Vocational Rehabilitation Programs for the Disabled: National Long Term Follow Up Study," *Social Security Bulletin*, Vol. 38, No. 10 (1975), p. 10.

20. Frederick C. Collignon and Richard Dodson, *Benefit-Cost Analysis of Vocational Rehabilitation Services Provided to Individuals Most Severely Handicapped* (Berkeley, Calif.: Berkeley Planning Associates, 1975), p. 14.

21. Abt Associates, pp. 196–201.

22. Abt Associates, pp. 167, 249.

23. U.S., General Accounting Office, *Effectiveness of Vocational Rehabilitation*, p. 30.

24. Abt Associates, pp. 233–234.

25. These studies are summarized and standardized in Disability and Health Economics Research Section, Bureau of Economic Research, *An Evaluation of the Structure and Function of Disability Programs*, Year 1 Summary Report (New Brunswick, N.J.: Rutgers University, 1975), pp. 188–196.

26. U.S., General Accounting Office, *Effectiveness of Vocational Rehabilitation*.

27. U.S., Department of Health, Education, and Welfare, Rehabilitation Services Administration, Division of Disability Studies, Office of Research and Statistics, "Work Adjustment of the Recently Disabled," *Disability Survey 71: Recently Disabled Adults*, Report No. 3, by Edward Steinberg (January 1976), Table 1-5.

28. Joe Nay, John Scanlon, and Joseph S. Wholey, *Benefits and Costs of Manpower Training Programs: A Synthesis of Previous Studies with Reservations and Recommendations* (Washington, D.C.: The Urban Institute, 1971), p. 11.

148 ALTERNATIVES IN REHABILITATING THE HANDICAPPED

29. These studies are carefully analyzed in U.S., National Commission on State Workmen's Compensation, "A Review of Benefit-Cost Analysis in Vocational Rehabilitation," *Supplemental Studies for the National Commission on State Workmen's Compensation Laws*, Vol. II., Study No. 21, by Larry L. Kiser (Washington, D.C.: U.S. Government Printing Office, 1973), pp. 383–396.
30. Disability and Health Economics Research Section, Bureau of Economic Research.
31. Collignon and Dodson.
32. Abt Associates, p. 260.
33. U.S., Department of Labor, Employment and Training Administration, "Changes in the Duration of Post Training Period in Relative Earnings Credits of Trainees," unpublished report by David J. Farber, August 1971.
34. Greenblum, p. 10.
35. U.S., Congress, House, Committee on Ways and Means, *Committee Staff Report on the Disability Insurance Program*, 93rd Cong., 2d sess., 1974, pp. 303–304.
36. U.S., Congress, House, Committee on Ways and Means, pp. 303–304.
37. U.S., Congress, House, Committee on Ways and Means, pp. 303–304.
38. U.S., General Accounting Office, *Improvements Needed in Efforts to Rehabilitate Social Security Disability Insurance Beneficiaries* (Washington, D.C.: U.S. Government Printing Office, 1975).
39. Monroe Berkowitz, William G. Johnson, and Edward H. Murphy, *Measuring the Effects of Disability on Work and Transfer Payments* (New Brunswick, N.J.: Bureau of Economic Research, Disability and Health Economics Research Section, Rutgers University, 1972), pp. 188–196.
40. Donald M. Bellante, "A Multivariate Analysis of a Vocational Rehabilitation Program," *The Journal of Human Resources*, Vol. 7, No. 2 (1972), p. 230.
41. Disability and Health Economics Research Section, Bureau of Economic Research, pp. 328–339.
42. Ronald Conley, "A Benefit/Cost Analysis of the Vocational Rehabilitation Program," *Journal of Human Resources*, Vol. 4, No. 2 (1969), p. 249.
43. Bellante, pp. 236–240.
44. Disability and Health Economics Research Section, Bureau of Economic Research, p. 342.

45. U.S. DHEW, RSA, *Agency Program Data, Fiscal Year 1975*, pp. 2–30.
46. U.S. DHEW, RSA, *Agency Program Data, Fiscal Year 1975*, pp. 2–30.
47. U.S. DHEW, RSA, *Agency Program Data, Fiscal Year 1975*, pp. 2–30.
48. U.S., Department of Health, Education, and Welfare, Rehabilitation Services Administration, *Caseload Statistics, State Vocational Rehabilitation Agencies, 1973* (Washington, D.C.: U.S. Government Printing Office, 1974), p. 11.
49. U.S., Department of Health, Education, and Welfare, Social Security Administration, *1972 Survey of the Disabled*, unpublished tabulations.
50. U.S., General Accounting Office, *Improvements Needed*; and U.S., Congress, House, Committee on Ways and Means, pp. 275–315.
51. Monroe Berkowitz, William G. Johnson, and Edward H. Murphy, *Public Policy Toward Disability* (New York: Praeger, 1976).
52. National Commission on State Workmen's Compensation, *Compendium on Workmen's Compensation* (Washington, D.C.: U.S. Government Printing Office, 1973), p. 162.

Chapter 3

VOCATIONAL REHABILITATION PERSPECTIVES FOR POLICY ANALYSIS AND CHANGE

Marvin B. Sussman

THE ISSUES

The development of appropriate policies for vocational rehabilitation requires consideration of four issues. The first issue arises because of the position of vocational rehabilitation within the context of a larger human service system of health and rehabilitation care. In devising program strategies, policymakers must inquire into the nature of the constraints that this larger system imposes on vocational rehabilitation practice. A second issue concerns the definition and measurement of disability. Disability has been conceived of as a medical condition or as a complex physical, social, and psychological process; how disability is defined will have a marked influence on the direction and objectives of the rehabilitation program. The third policy issue centers on the question of the most appropriate "unit" for rehabilitation treatment: should rehabilitation efforts be geared toward the disabled individual alone or toward the family as a whole? The final issue has emerged recently because of changes in the relationship of professionals and clients. Policymakers must consider whether the traditional superordinate-subordinate model of rehabilitation should be replaced by the parity model of shared authority and shared responsibility.

In the first section of this chapter, I will examine each of these issues in greater detail. The inquiry is intended to clarify the rationales for, and objectives of, rehabilitation policy, and to serve as a necessary preliminary step to the presentation of specific program recommendations in the second section.

Human Service System Constraints

An important consideration for policymakers is that many individuals have only limited access to available health resources. Most often denied are the poor, members of ethnic and racial minorities, the elderly, and "difficult" cases.[1] Even though the majority of the health and rehabilitation facilities are found in urban areas, many residents in need of health and rehabilitation services do not receive them. A recent study in Tennessee of over 12,000 inner city families indicated that only 13 percent of those requiring medical care were receiving it.[2]

The findings of the 1972 Survey of Disabled and Nondisabled Adults suggest that the problem of access to care is one which the disabled share with other individuals in need of health services:

> About 1 in 5 of the severely disabled said that they did not try to get services because they did not know of available services. This is a somewhat greater proportion than reported by the partially disabled. This group of over 1 million severely disabled adults who said they did not know of services may have contained many who might have benefited from services.[3]

About 900,000 of the disabled, 600,000 of those who were "currently" disabled at the time of the study and 300,000 recovered disabled, reported that their efforts to obtain rehabilitation services were unsuccessful. Lack of qualification (15 percent) and no agency response (20 percent) were the reasons for no service given by the 300,000 severely disabled in the study.[4]

Multiple reasons are probable as to why access to rehabilitation services is denied or limited to certain individuals and groups of different cultural backgrounds, ages, and types and degrees of disability. The procedures that applicants must undergo to be declared eligible for services are complex, and agencies may be biased in their selection of clients by their desire to obtain maximal successful outcomes. The current system of disseminating information about rehabilitation services, options, and entitlements may also be inadequate.

Another problem related to the provision of quality medical and rehabilitation services is its increasing high cost. While the overall dollars spent for such services may have increased as a result of rapidly growing demand, the overwhelming reasons for the dollar increase are inflation and the high labor cost for such services. In 1975, $118 billion was spent for health care services, an amount that constitutes approximately 8.3 percent of the gross national product.[5] Medicare and Medicaid programs, upon which so many persons who are disabled or retired depend, are providing fewer benefits and are costing more because of inflation and labor cost increases.[6] The situation is not improved when a sudden rise in unemployment occurs as was the case in 1975. Citizens who lose their jobs soon after lost their health and insurance coverage.[7] Consequences were increased demands on existing public systems to provide the necessary social and welfare services, medical care, and rehabilitation.

Monies spent for federal-state vocational rehabilitation were $30 million in 1950, $165 million in 1965, and $809 million in 1974.[8] Monroe Berkowitz, William Johnson, and Edward Murphy studied the interrelationship between cash transfers, medical payments, and direct services, a trinity of functions to restore a maximum number of disabled persons to an independent living status. If independence is equated with return to gainful employment, then a direct service program (vocational rehabilitation) is indicated, with appropriate medical care and cash transfers to cover purchase of medical services and maintenance during the rehabilitation regimen. If independence is interpreted as the individual's ability to perform activities of daily living (ADL) then cash transfer becomes a high priority, and services and ADL instruction play a secondary role. The Berkowitz team focused on cash transfers from all sources and indicated the following trend:

> Total transfers increased by 96% between 1967 and 1973, and by 116% at the federal level during the same space of time. In real terms, after adjusting for inflation, transfer payments in 1973 were 47% greater than in 1967, and at the federal level the increase was 63%. Using a different measure of disability—transfer payments limited to those ages 18–64—we estimate that since 1967, transfers have been increasing about 9% per year. If such trends continue, transfers will amount to nearly $115 billion in constant 1967 dollars by 1980.[9]

These cost data suggest increasing resistance to further appropriations and new programs.

Even if individuals have the money to pay for health services, they may have difficulty entering the health care system. Specialization within the medical field and the shortage of physicians who practice in primary care areas (less than one-third of all physicians) contribute to fragmentation and deficiencies in the delivery of health services.[10] In addition, little effort has been expended to integrate medical and rehabilitation services, largely because the geographical distribution of health and rehabilitation facilities would make such integration difficult. Problems in obtaining integrated medical and rehabilitation services may inhibit the implementation of a policy and program based on a holistic concept of medical and rehabilitation objectives. Policies and programs to develop a team approach in the delivery of such services, however, will be further explored in this chapter.

Another critical issue is that a large number of Americans, approximately 41,000,000 under retirement age, do not have any health insurance, and twice as many blacks as whites lack coverage for hospitalization and medical services.[11] Existing insurance is uneven in coverage and lacks uniform standards or criteria that will provide maximal protection for the client. One author has noted that such features of insurance policies as deductibles, co-insurance and uncovered services make coverage more an "illusion than reality."[12] For those individuals who will actually need vocational rehabilitation, entry into the health care system is problematic and sometimes impossible. With such variation in coverage, we might also expect that quality of service will vary greatly in relation to cost and availability of monies to pay for services.

Another issue, which is threatening what little stability exists today in the medical and rehabilitation system, is the effort by consumers, social innovators, intellectuals, and some practitioners to make the availability of services a matter of right rather than eligibility. These groups seriously question the current ideologies behind medical and rehabilitation care; they take the position that individuals are entitled to services and should be allowed a more active role in the design of those services.

The movement towards client participation in activities related to their health and rehabilitation received significant government support through an April 1975 Presidential directive. The directive was intended to improve consumer representation in government decision making, and it called for the development of an appropriate organizational mechanism for consumer affairs, increased consumer representation in government bureaus and advisory councils, consumer input into the decision-making process, and the provision to the public of specialized consumer information and educational programs for consumer responsibility. The directive also indicated that an evaluation program should be created to handle consumer complaints and to work toward the development of new policies and service programs.

In November 1975, Consumer Representation Plans for all federal agencies were submitted to the President of the United States.[13] A number of strategies for improving consumer representation were included in the plans, and some agencies seriously considered adopting an ombudsman model. The Department of Health, Education, and Welfare, which has historically sought a high degree of consumer representation, expressed its intention to handle consumer complaints more efficiently and to evaluate these in relation to necessary policy and program modifications. The Social Security Administration (SSA) indicated a desire to experiment with the ombudsman concept to handle those grievances of beneficiaries which demand an immediate solution.

The implementation of such plans may have a twofold effect: the protection of client interests and the concomitant reduction of the authority and power of the provider. It is also likely that the plans will prove to be a catalyst in the movement to uphold "service rights" over the notion of restricted eligibility based on socioeconomic criteria or functional limitation. While it is impossible to predict the long-range effects of the plans with any certainty, it is clear that the current policies of disability management and rehabilitation, and the principles upon which they operate, are now open to challenge.

As part of the human service system, then, vocational rehabilitation and other services for the disabled share in both the advances and the shortcomings of the field. The problems of limited access to health care, rapidly increasing costs, and poorly integrated services confront those persons who suffer from chronic, as well as acute, illnesses and impairments. But the disabled have also benefitted along with other groups from such broad developments as the consumer advocacy and clients' rights movements.

One further way in which the human service system as a whole has affected vocational rehabilitation is in the attitudes toward rehabilitation that it engenders among the disabled. In the 1972 Survey of Disabled and Nondisabled Adults, 4 in 10 of the "currently disabled" respondents and 8 in 10 of the "no longer disabled" respondents indicated that they did not seek rehabilitation services because they "didn't need any."[14] Undoubtedly for some or even a large proportion of the disabled respondents this assessment is a just one. Their injuries may not be severe and they will not require rehabilitation services to return to their former job or to a similar job. There is, however, a group of disabled individuals who reject services because of human service system constraints. Although they might benefit from services, they adopt the posture of "didn't need any" or "doubted it could help." Such a response may stem from misperception of need, or it may reflect an individual's skepticism about the value of services or his own ability to obtain and profit by such services. It may also grow out of a form of client "inertia" or apathy. What is significant is that attitudes of this kind can, in fact, be fostered by the rehabilitation system itself. Rehabilitation clients become members of a social category, "recipients of services," soon after entering the system. They quickly assimilate the beliefs and values of this group in which they hold membership. While client-centered groups can promote positive attitudes and expectations, they can also have the opposite effect, helping to create a climate of pessimism and apathy.

Other findings of the 1972 Survey may throw light on the question of client dissatisfaction with rehabilitation services. A significant number of the respondents indicated that job training and placement, or activities directly related to reentry into the labor market, were of higher interest than physical therapy and special devices.[15] Because physical, medical, and psychological therapies are often the necessary preliminary steps to job training and placement, these data might be interpreted to mean that many clients desire to go beyond the maintenance therapies. The data might also suggest that rehabilitation of the disabled typically halts when a maintenance level is reached.

Policymakers should take the 1972 survey response into consideration in evaluating the rehabilitation system and in formulating new approaches to rehabilitation. Methods of overcoming client indifference and of guarding against the possibility of misperceived needs should be investigated, and a more ambitious program of vocational and placement services might be adopted. Finally, agencies of the system should be responsible for informing their clientele, promptly and candidly, of the constraints under which they operate and the nature of their professional competencies and deficits. Clients and potential clients should have a realistic understanding of what the vocational rehabilitation system can and cannot do.

Changing Meanings and Definitions of Rehabilitation and Its Components

A second important issue concerns the definition and measurement of disability. For many years, the term *disability* was interpreted differently to suit the varied needs of program administrators, government officials, and medical personnel. Now however, there is a movement toward the adoption of uniform definitions. Emergent entitlement policies, contracts between providers and clients, and ombudsmanship systems have figured in this movement. So too has the seminal work of Saad Nagi, *Disability and Rehabilitation: Legal, Clinical and Self Concepts and Measurement*, which established important distinctions between impairment, disability, handicap, and severity. Nagi defined *impairment* as some anatomic or physiologic loss expressed as a physical or mental deficit, e.g., memory loss, absence of a limb, hearing loss, paralysis of lower limbs; he defined *disability* as a limitation in functioning caused by an impairment, such as limitations in walking, sitting, reading, working, or interacting with others. *Handicaps* are limitations in the individual's ability to carry on expected activities such as performing competently in school or work, or taking care of one's personal needs; and *severity* is the degree of impairment, disability, or handicap.[16]

As definitions of concepts go, these are reasonably concise. However, problems arise when these concepts are put into practice. How does one measure limitations? What are the criteria for determining the degree of severity? These definitional problems bothered rehabilitation staff members, representatives in the Congress, and consultants preparing the 1973 rehabilitation bill that would ensure delivery of services to the most severely handicapped. Eventually, the Congress rejected as a measure of severity the effects of the handicap on costs and time of rehabilitation. It chose instead a categorical approach, using the cause of the handicap to define the group under issue.

While the Congressional decision represented a return to a conservative measure of disability, legislation during the 1960s tended to expand the definition of "the disabled" to include the socially and culturally disadvantaged. The use of these expanded definitions helped to transform the rehabilitation program from a personal counseling model to a sociopsychological one. William Gellman describes this new rehabilitation:

> Rehabilitation becomes a community-centered program reaching into the cultures of the poor, disabled and disadvantaged. Clients are seen as participants rather than recipients. Services include all types of techniques which can move clients toward productive work. The most important service is provision of a concrete goal accessible to all clients—work in a non-competitive work system developed by rehabilitation and providing work to all rehabilitatees regardless of productive level. Given this type of work system, all clients can achieve some degree of success in the rehabilitation process.[17]

One can disagree with Gellman that employment in a non-competitive work situation is a desired goal of rehabilitation, while still accepting the viability of a successful community-based rehabilitation system for the poor and disenfranchised. Return to gainful employment in competitive jobs is the preferred goal. Protective jobs such as those provided by government public works programs are a less desirable alternative, a fall-back if the job market cannot absorb the rehabilitee. Gellman may be more of a realist than those who hold the position that job placement in competitive positions is the only justifiable objective of rehabilitation. He foresees a group of able-bodied and disabled who will never be successfully absorbed into the work force because of conditions endemic to a free enterprise economy. Foremost among these conditions are chronic job shortages, inappropriate education and training of workers, and the constraints imposed by an advancing technology and by the rules of such organizations as corporations and unions.

The acceptance of rehabilitation as a major tool to overcome long-term dependence and the extension of the program to serve new groups of clients will require new definitions of successful outcome. Definitions of acceptable outcomes will not only come from professionals in rehabilitation but increasingly from clients and their advocates.

It is doubtful that a policy providing comprehensive services without vocational goals will be or even should be effected in the foreseeable future. The implications are that the severely handicapped, given priority to enter the rehabilitation system, may be washed out before admission, even with provisions that comprehensive services be extended to applicants who presently could not be judged to have a vocational goal. In clarification of the regulatory statutes, the Rehabilitation Services Administration emphasized that the purpose of such services is to bring the handicapped person to the point where a vocational goal is feasible and rehabilitation could commence. The statutory intent does not eliminate the requirements for the establishment of vocational objectives and achievement of vocational goals for the handicapped person served by its agencies, even with the mandated priority to provide services to severely handicapped persons.

With monies scarce for comprehensive (prevocational rehabilitation training) services under Title I, Part C of the PL 93-112, and with the Rehabilitation Services Administration's careful emphasis on establishing and achieving vocational goals and objectives, it is unlikely that many severely disabled persons will enter and move through the system and into the world of work. The apparent contradictions in our policy toward the rehabilitation of the severely disabled invited speculation that nonvocational or alternative rehabilitation goals will become a legitimate program objective when the statistical record becomes available a few years hence.

While varied definitions and determinants of eligibility for rehabilitation may constrain entry into the system, there are some indications that clients are taking on increased responsibility for their own well-being. The number of client social organizations is growing. The clients' rights movements are becoming more active and finding support for their goals in the consumerism movement and in recent federal legislation. Professional providers are coming to the recognition that in "treating" an individual, whether it is for a health, rehabilitation, or welfare problem, it is worthwhile to treat a larger group of intimates, particularly the members of the individual's household. By dealing with a family or household group, providers have a better chance of effecting lasting positive outcomes, often at reduced cost.

Family or Household as Unit of Rehabilitation

Family sociologists, social psychologists, and anthropologists have established that human beings, for the most part, live and function in primary groups such as families. Human beings depend upon such groups for their emotional, and to a large degree their physical, survival from childhood on. It is a group that provides needed affection, intimacy, bonding, and shared tasks and responsibilities; it enables the individual to learn his or her identity and roles in order to be able to function in the larger society. Most groups are hierarchically organized and the individual is controlled, or at least influenced, by those who have been given power or have themselves achieved power. In the case of voluntary associations, the person's perceptions, attitudes, values, and, ultimately, behaviors are influenced by those who have achieved position and status within the group. In the family, children are, of course, influenced by their parents. While this influence may ebb in time, the early socialization establishes lifetime values, behaviors, and relationships. The significance of these primary group relationships has been confirmed by several empirical studies that show that the overwhelming majority of individuals will opt for family relationships if these are at all possible.[18]

The family is given the major legal responsibility for its members and is asked to handle the problems of its "deviant" and dependent. Even though we have established human service systems unmatched in cost and magnitude by any other country in past or contemporary history, it is the family that is principally accountable for the care and well-being of its members throughout their lives.

Many individuals find that their "everyday family" is most significant to them in relation to how they feel, perceive, think, and behave. The everyday family has been characterized as the group with whom one identifies; its members may or may not be related by blood or marriage, but they are essentially one's intimates—persons one goes to when in trouble, persons one likes to be with. These individuals provide motivation, understanding, friendship, and pleasure.[19] Such primary groups give purpose and meaning to individual lives and are undoubtedly the most important networks for the estimated 20 percent of the U.S. population who are currently single and living alone or in communal arrangements.[20]

The pluralistic family structure has considerable significance for vocational rehabilitation.[21] In treating individuals who have a disability, the rehabilitation system is actually engaging a group, in most instances, a family. Because the problems of family members are ultimately relegated to the family, as both legal and moral responsibilities, disability and rehabilitation is a family concern. How the rehabilitation client responds to the system, maintains a level of motivation sufficient to complete the rehabilitation regimen, and pursues his or her vocational objectives will be a function of his or her participation in the family group. The group's acceptance of the individual's disability, their willingness to act as a buffer between the individual and the provider system, the impact of disability upon all family members, and finally, the disabled member's role and status within the family are factors that will influence the individual's rehabilitation experience and its outcome. As time passes, the entire family system will increasingly be viewed as the natural key to the effective functioning of an individual member who has come to be labelled "disabled." From the client's perspective, the family is critical for survival and for reaching and maintaining gains from rehabilitation, whether these are optimal mobility, performance of the activities of daily living, or holding a job.

Persons who have recently experienced an illness or injury and are placed in a care or treatment system in which they have little input or control are more likely to have lowered self-concepts than the non-ill or injured. While some disabled persons express anger and hostility and fight the system, the overwhelming majority take on the role of being the "good" patient by conforming. Unless the system provides meaningful and warm relationships for the client, the only available option is to turn to one's family or friends for support and understanding. In all fairness, treatment institutions and service agencies are not organized to provide extensive emotional and social supports; the training of professionals and related service personnel to be competent in such matters is a fairly new procedure. Moreover, it is usually assumed that the family will act upon its legal and moral responsibility to look after its own. Where the family does not exist, the substitute primary group, e.g., household or intimate friendship group, often does the caretaking and supporting based on a nonlegal group norm of reciprocation. Friends and relatives who are close are expected to respond when one is in need, and the significant test of the relationship is in the response.

Many individuals who experience crises such as divorce, accident, acute illness, or a chronic condition, in time become alienated and experience a loss of self-control. Such persons depend upon others for support and affection at the same time they need to be motivated to help themselves.[22] In a study of workers' compensation cases in five states, William G. Johnson and Julia Makarushka of Syracuse University measured the level of alienation and self-control of claimants. On an average, 53 percent of all workers' compensation claimants agreed with the statement, "no one can be found to count on," and 52.8 percent agreed with the statement, "most people don't care about others."[23] Undoubtedly, some claimants in answering these questions included members of their families among those who were unaccountable and unconcerned. It would be naive to assume that all family members respond enthusiastically to the responsibilities of caring for ill or disabled members over long periods of time. Chronic illness and disability can place unexpected pressures on marital relationships, and there is some evidence that troubled marriages tend to dissolve after such serious health crises occur.[24]

The client's need for support to reduce feelings of alienation and to restore a sense of future prospects for a good life still persists regardless of the family situation. How to strengthen the family by providing incentives and social supports is a matter that is taken up in a second section of the chapter. A method of making the family part of the provider system, working in collaboration with medical and rehabilitation agencies, is also presented.

How one is treated while under medical care and rehabilitation is related to alienation and lowered self-esteem and the need for response from intimates. Two questions concerned with satisfaction and fair treatment were posed to respondents in the Syracuse study. First, the investigators asked the respondents to evaluate their rehabilitation experience. They then divided the responses into four categories: very satisfied, little satisfied, little dissatisfied, and very dissatisfied. The investigators found that 26.2 percent of claimants receiving rehabilitation in the five states indicated some level of dissatisfaction with the services provided.

A second survey question concerned fair treatment under the workers' compensation program. Johnson and Makarushka categorized the question along three dimensions: whether the claimant was treated "very fairly" when compared with other cases, "somewhat fairly," or "not fairly." Almost 30 percent of the respondents indicated that they were not fairly treated. Being "somewhat fairly treated," if not an ambivalent response, is at least not a very enthusiastic one, and 36.4 percent of workers' compensation claimants responded in this manner. Thirty-four percent of all respondents indicated they were very fairly treated when compared with other claimants. The rank order of fairness by states was Wisconsin, 43 percent; New York, 37 percent; Florida, 34 percent; Washington, 31 percent; and California, 25 percent.

Data collected by Cooper and Company and by Johnson and Makarushka furnish evidence that there is some impact upon the family as a consequence of a work-related injury or disability.[25] The questions that these researchers asked of workers' compensation claimants did not specifically address possible changes in the patterns of family relationships because of injury or disability. However, a sizable number of claimants indicated that they now required support and sought help from family members. The necessity for other family members to enter the work force in order to compensate for wage losses implies that internal changes in roles and interaction patterns are occurring. One can assume that in those situations where a female partner was entering the work force for the first time, she was undertaking significant new responsibilities, even if her relationship with the disabled person was not greatly modified. Her feelings about working, about continuing to perform household tasks, or as an alternative, shifting those tasks to others, could affect the claimant's ability to enter rehabilitation and to recoup the psychological, occupational, and financial losses usually associated with injury and illness.

The Cooper Company interviewers asked each claimant whether family members had to go to work as a consequence of his or her injury or illness. For the four reporting states, New York, California, Illinois, and Georgia, 14 percent of the compensated cases indicated that family members had entered the work force. Claimants reported that a family member had to enter gainful employment in 50 percent of the noncompensated cases in California and 43 percent in Georgia. In California, the ratio of noncompensated to compensated cases was 0.13 and in Georgia it was 0.9.

The Johnson and Makarushka study indirectly addressed the need for a postinjury family adjustment by asking respondents who had gone through the workers' compensation system whether their spouses had to change their work patterns a year after the injury occurred; 17 percent in Wisconsin, 18 percent in New York, 19 percent in California, 24 percent in Florida, and 36 percent in Washington made occupational transitions. The mean for all five states was 22.8 percent; in more than one in five families, the claimant's partner underwent a change in jobs or career. [26]

Workers who are injured or become ill and qualify as a claimant are concerned initially about becoming healthy once again, and fortunately this is also the major emphasis of those in charge of health and rehabilitation systems. The normal process is to restore the health of the worker in order to minimize the consequences of the impairment, which may be the result of, or concomitant with, the disability, and then to proceed to rehabilitation. The issue is whether claimants said they needed help in household work and such other chores as meal preparation, and what persons or agencies the claimants turned to as a source of help. Respondents in the Johnson and Makarushka study responded in the affirmative (20.2 percent) when asked whether they needed help from someone because of health reasons. Californians and Washingtonians expressed greater need for help (29.6 percent and 27.0 percent, respectively) than residents of Florida (15.6 percent), New York (11.3 percent), and Wisconsin (17.5 percent). Very few respondents indicated that they would seek help from an agency person for personal care or household tasks; most relied upon obtaining assistance from their spouses or children. Friends also respond when the individual needs this form of help. Family members, especially spouses, and to a lesser degree relatives and friends, help the disabled individuals in the activities of daily living. The responses suggest that claimants find friends and family reliable, but are not inclined to seek assistance from agencies for personal- and home-oriented activities.

In general, the "not married" respondents, consisting of the widowed, separated, and divorced, tended to feel a need for help from children approximately as much as, and in some states more than, those married. Ironically, this group is far more likely to receive help from other relatives.

In seeking such assistance, the injured, ill, or disabled person develops various dependencies upon other family members and relatives. In responding to these needs, the family or primary group must expend and reallocate the limited resources of income, time, and energy available to it. The quality of life that these family members will experience, and in some situations their very survival, will be dependent upon the competencies that they develop to handle the new situation. They must sustain a high level of motivation, and create the type of conditions that will enable them to achieve some self-determined life-style. The fortunes of the injured or disabled individual, moreover, are interwoven with those of the family or household unit and the individual's ability to adapt will depend in large measure upon theirs. Currently, the extensive network of service programs is geared primarily to assist the individual and does not give sufficient consideration to the personal, social, and economic impact upon the family or household. This network also overlooks the family or household as a potential contributor to the rehabilitation of its disabled member.

Return to the work force after disability is more likely if individuals are married, and if the spouse is supportive and assisting.[27] Marital status not only influences work force participation, but also positively affects the actual number of hours worked.[28] These findings are in consonance with the established predictor of labor force participation, namely, being married and living with one's spouse.[29]

Health and marital status are also correlated; disabled individuals who are married are less susceptible to mental illnesses and personality disorders. Because being married is associated both with a return to the work force and with the ability to maintain mental health at higher levels than the nonmarried, interest has arisen in the consequences of intrafamily dynamics for rehabilitation outcomes. Economists such as Berkowitz, Johnson, and Murphy, using their own analytic methods, have reached conclusions similar to those obtained by other social scientists:

> The basic importance of marital status as an indicator of labor force behavior is not much diminished by our discovery of small but significant second-order relationships between marital status and health. It is worth noting that the reasons for the observed importance of marital status for both impaired and nonimpaired workers are not well understood. Financial considerations aside, the attitudes and activities of other household members would seem to be essential determinants of the reaction of an individual to the limiting effects of impairment. A better knowledge of these attitudes and interactions would improve public policy decisions concerning the type and amount of family-directed services offered by rehabilitation and welfare agencies. The effects of transfer payment programs' eligibility criteria and payment levels on family structure could also be more clearly understood.
>
> It seems that the obvious and familiar importance of marital status as an influence on labor supply may lead investigators to overlook the reasons for its importance and its special relationship to the problem of disability. Its peculiar association with mental illness and the more powerful relation between it and the disability status of impaired persons deserve additional study.[30]

Ideally, the role played by family and friendship groups in the rehabilitation process will grow as the rehabilitation system itself evolves. Today, many rehabilitation clients, counselors and administrators are skeptical about the ability of traditional organizational and training procedures to effect satisfactory rehabilitation outcomes. These individuals are seeking more productive and less costly rehabilitation options. Clearly, the strategy of assigning families an important role in the rehabilitation process is one possibility that merits consideration.

Recent Changes in Client-Practitioner Relations and Implications for Rehabilitation Practices

The complex bureaucracy behind human services delivery has standardized rehabilitation regulations and procedures to such an extent that clients are seeking more personalized care and questioning the power and expertise of professional caretakers. Clients are demanding that human service system professionals discuss the service options with them in advance and that both parties work out a contract that will ensure delivery of the services that the client selects and maximize the client's chances of achieving his or her rehabilitation goals. A brief review of the development of rehabilitation programs will serve to illustrate the real importance of establishing better communication between clients and program personnel.

The growth of the rehabilitation system in the United States has occurred largely under government sponsorship. The rehabilitation profession was in effect created with the passage of legislation after World War I and is practiced largely in government settings. In the post-World War II period, the concept of the team approach was introduced,[31] and the population served was expanded to include all the handicapped. The federal government subsidized the training of more specialists to encourage their entrance into the field, and rehabilitation rapidly became a highly professionalized, interdisciplinary program. Predictably, the growth in the number of practitioners was accompanied by a growth in the number of administrators, and a complex bureaucratic structure came into being to oversee the rehabilitation operations. J. P. Zelle described this development:

> When the counselor of a few years past was a sort of general practitioner to the vocationally handicapped, he was able to work with rather simple and understandable jurisdictions. His modern counterpart tends more and more to be specialized and integrated

into large multidisciplinary institutional work settings. Here diverse split-off options cause role and jurisdictional confusions with other vocations in the behavioral science field.[32]

While some view the interdisciplinary team approach of rehabilitation as an obvious strength of the field,[33] others suggest that the plethora of professionals creates unnecessary overlapping and duplication in the provision of services.[34] Similarly, many view the professionalization of rehabilitation occupations unfavorably. T. P. Hipkins, for example, writes:

> There seems to have been a need immediately upon emergence for the fledgling professions to build defenses to protect the new-won territory from intrusion by others. In the process we have developed "professional standards and ethics" whose original intent was to raise the quality of care to those needing it. But, as in almost every emerging profession, it has materialized too often as a device for insuring the profession's self-preservation first and quality care to people later—maybe—are we really talking about standards or ethics or quality or are we really talking about restraint of trade?[35]

Richard Hardy and Keith Wright are even more negative in their assessment of the impact of these developments on rehabilitation:

> Rehabilitation is splintered in goals, settings, services and professional groups. There should be a mutual trust toward what might be called "applied rehabilitation," or dealing with the human service story rather than debating about professional integrity and rank ordering disciplines. We have become so highly involved with licensing, certification, specialization, and professionalization that we have extended enormous amounts of energy building for ourselves professional kingdoms over which to reign. These efforts, in some cases, have thus dissipated our energies and weakened our frontal attack on the problems of the society—those of handicapping conditions.[36]

Similarly, Paul Ellwood suggests that the separate turfs maintained by each profession in rehabilitation lead to loss of time, increased costs, and inconvenience. The findings of these authors point to a need for reducing the degree of specialization in the field of rehabilitation.

Client assertiveness may prove to be one remedy for the problems that the authors cite. As clients seek a greater measure of control over the rehabilitation process, they may counteract the tendency of the whole system to expand "at the top." By questioning current rehabilitation practices and priorities and by demanding certain reforms, clients may regain some of the authority that now rests with the program's professional and administrative superstructure.

The "client rebellion" began in the 1960s with opposition to authority and the presumption of expertise, an opposition that is still continuing.[37] Clients challenged the traditional superordinate-subordinate model of the relationship between the provider and the client in the human service sector. Patients and clients began to demand parity relationships and collateral decision making. Heightened concern with entitlements to service, professional accountability, and contractual treatment put an additional strain on the traditional professional client relationship. Client organizations and client advocates or ombudsmen emerged as influential forces in the already complex rehabilitation arena. All of the efforts by clients to achieve a greater degree of participation in the rehabilitation process were collectively labelled "client assertiveness."

Assertiveness could take a number of forms: the client might object to a treatment or rehabilitation arrangement in which he or she is expected to accept most of the provider's values and attitudes; to assume the role of status inferior in the relationship; to be receptive to various forms of behavior modification; to have very little or no say in the decisions concerning treatment; or to make few efforts to resist control by the professional.[38] What clients have reacted against is the superordinate-subordinate model of professional-client interaction, where learning is in one direction only, flowing from the professional to the client.

Client assertiveness began with efforts at self-organization and representation. The boot camp training in socialization took place on the wards.[39] Patient or family clubs, welfare mothers' groups, client membership in hospital boards of directors, and ombudsman groups are examples of current organizational forms.

In the late 1960s, client assertiveness reached a mature stage. Client groups who had begun by demonstrating in the streets became, to a large extent, respectable and institutionalized. Those groups concerned with rehabilitation now seek involvement at all levels of the rehabilitation process. They help to determine the needs of the disabled and disadvantaged, assist in the provision of services and the administration of programs, participate in program evaluation, and work in the neglected area of follow-up care.[40]

Today's client groups are working on strategies that go far beyond marches and protests. They seek to be effective lobbyists, to influence legislators, and to move public opinion. In this way, they hope to generate widespread support for their objectives, to affect public policy and the allocation of public funds, and more specifically to bring about the program changes which they desire. The May 1977 "march" to Washington by the severely disabled resulted in immediate action by the Secretary of Health, Education and Welfare on the guidelines governing implementation of equal opportunity provisions for the severely disabled. The march is only one indicator of the capacity of the client groups to exercise political power.

The movement toward client self-actualization has been supported by a large number of "new" professionals. These professionals grew up in the countercultures of the 1960s and are now leading their peers and senior colleagues in bringing medicine, health care, and rehabilitation back into the community and the home.

For example, family medicine, which takes a holistic approach to disease causality, diagnosis, and treatment, is no longer a low-status clinical specialty but is receiving substantial governmental financial aid and acceptance by the American Medical Association, physicians and patients.

> While the physician is functioning in a 'jack-of-all-trades' role, he is being perceived by the patient less as a meddler and more as a collaborator-expert. These new devotees of a reciprocal model of patient-professional relationship are still too few to signify a complete remodeling of current medical care and rehabilitation delivery systems. But the handwriting is on the wall. The traditional rehabilitation and health care system no longer has the ideological supports, or even political muscle, to maintain its established position.[41]

Human service professionals have revived the ancient and honored Scandinavian practice of representation by ombudsman, although they have modified it to some extent to suit the ethos and values of our society. Historically, an ombudsman represented the government or the company management and handled worker grievances. His modern counterpart, however, is answerable to a different party; no longer a company or government official, the ombudsman today serves as a client advocate and representative of client interests.

The emergence of advocacy groups has helped to make the client an equal partner with the practitioner in the rehabilitation process. Similarly, recent legislation that sets forth the basis of a "contract" arrangement will undoubtedly lead to a greater degree of reciprocity in the relations of the two parties. In the Rehabilitation Act of 1973, Section 102 provided major legislative support for a "people oriented" rehabilitation. In its original form, the provision called for the creation of a patient advocacy system and specified that one percent of the total rehabilitation budget be appropriated for patient's rights and advocacy. The final legislation did not contain this provision. Too many members of the House of Representatives were fearful that radicals might take over the client cause, and they associated such a provision with the one that funded community development programs during the "War on Poverty" period and that gave rise to a new group of black and other minority politicians in the urban ghettoes.

In its final form, Section 102 of the Rehabilitation Act of 1973 required an individualized rehabilitation program for eligible disabled persons under a broadening mandate. The planning of individualized rehabilitation regimens has been long in existence, but these regimens have been carried out with little client input and without guarantee of effective client and agency performance. Section 102 clearly indicates that rehabilitation clients, as well as all other citizens in their search for security and independence, should obtain services under the notion of entitlement. This was the view of the Congress and President in passing the 1973 legislation, and Section 102 provided a mechanism for enforcement of entitlement.

What are the implications of this legislation for the organization and delivery of rehabilitation services; for current client-practitioner relationships; and for the legal rights and obligations of clients, professionals, and rehabilitation agencies? These questions have recently come under investigation.

The individualized written client program is essentially a "contract," even if it is not legally defined as such. As with all agreements, it suggests implicit and explicit understandings; specifies rights and duties; establishes accountability; provides for evaluation of goals, procedures, and outcomes; promises fulfillment and compensation for breach; and calls for negotiation of terms. The essence of the contract is reciprocity, commitment, trust, and expectation. The notion of working together on a near parity basis towards a mutually agreed upon goal may require major changes in current rehabilitation ideologies and practices. Interpersonal relationships between clients, their families, and professionals will be affected, as will the organizational structure of the vocational rehabilitation program. The 1973 Act and subsequent amendments draw the rehabilitation program closer to a policy of service provision as a matter of entitlement, rather than a matter of agency or counselor discretion. The act also makes it possible for clients to achieve a greater understanding of their rights and responsibilities.

The notion of an "implicit" contract has existed in the rehabilitation field from the earliest days. In one sense, the contract facilitates the relationship. If it is a helping or treatment contract, such as the "individualized written rehabilitation program,"[42] then it should facilitate the helping process.

The importance of client inputs in the treatment process has been observed and documented by social and rehabilitation workers. Paul Abels, reporting on a study by Anne Shyne of clients served by a major Cleveland rehabilitation agency, has written, "it was found that one of the most frequent deterrents to continuance [of services] were differences of opinion between the worker and the client in the perception of the problem, and the worker's failure to help the client in a way that the client expected and wanted to be helped."[43] Abels also stresses the necessity of respecting client autonomy, i.e., the individual's control over his or her involvement in the rehabilitation program:

> The autonomy of the client is maintained when we are clearly able to (1) spell out the agency and worker function, (2) explore the range of decision-making open to both the client and the worker in this situation, (3) when we function in a manner which enables him to use his own decision-making resources, and (4) when we mutually agree on the goals and means of achieving them.[44]

By clarifying the expectations of the client and the professional, defining their respective decision-making powers, and setting forth the goals and means that have been mutually agreed upon, the contract may effect a change in the practices associated with the conventional model of rehabilitation. The possibility of modifying the superordinate-subordinate relationship in rehabilitation is probably a more significant consequence of the Rehabilitation Act of 1973 than the idea of contract as a legal form. A second contribution of the 1973 Act and the "individualized rehabilitation program" is its recognition that rehabilitation is a humanizing process and that successful rehabilitation depends as much upon the development of the client's social and interpersonal competence as upon the development of his job skills.

Individuals undergoing medical treatment and then entering

the rehabilitation system as clients are participants in a process. This process involves complex relationships with professionals, and practices that may be supportive or restrictive of client rehabilitation objectives. The Rehabilitation Act of 1973 signaled a new interest in evaluating the *process* of rehabilitation as well as specific rehabilitation outcomes. Concern is with the contribution of each component of the process to a set of objectives established by the patient or client with the professional. Philosophically, the shift is from a help system where professionals determine the services which clients will receive to one where clients are participating in all phases of the rehabilitation process. Here, professionals, clients, and family members are bonded together on the basis of trust and cooperation.

In review, the Rehabilitation Act of 1973 has the potential to alter the existing system of rehabilitation in a radical way. The Act can be seen as a move by the federal government to institutionalize client power. It may challenge the autonomy of professionals in the field and bring about substantial reforms in the rehabilitation programs in the coming decades.[45] The future development of vocational rehabilitation will clearly require careful monitoring.

Policy Recommendations

Family Dynamics and Family Mapping

The issue of the appropriate unit of rehabilitation treatment has been raised. Should rehabilitation efforts be directed toward the disabled individual alone, or toward his or her family and/or circle of intimates as well? Although it is customary for all human service providers to treat clients, patients and consumers as individuals, the effects of treatment, like the effects of disability itself, are felt by the entire "primary group." Conversely, the primary group will have a significant impact on the provider's efforts to improve the work competencies and skills of the disabled individual. The rehabilitation outcome will reflect the group's whole posture toward its disabled member—its rejection of him or her, on the one hand, or on the other, its acceptance and support.

In recognition of the important role played by the family in the rehabilitation process, policymakers might support the creation of a program to train rehabilitation staff in family structure and dynamics. Rehabilitation practitioners who underwent such training could be expected to explore diagnostic and treatment procedures which are family oriented, and perhaps to effect more successful rehabilitation outcomes. In order to attract professional interest, government might provide financial incentives to rehabilitation programs that include training in family dynamics and might make funds available for continuing education programs for professionals.

Policymakers might also consider the development of such practitioner tools as the "family diagnostic checklist." The list would record each claimant's most important relatives and relationships, as well as such factors as type of disability, age, sex, work history, and health status. The definition of family used in the checklist would be sociologic rather than legal; it would refer to the "everyday family" and include those persons considered to be "family" by the rehabilitee, as well as relations by blood or marriage. The diagnostic checklist would thus offer a comprehensive look at that group of individuals surrounding the rehabilitee who are bound to him by commitment, trust, intimacy, and affection but who do not necessarily live in the same household. The checklist would serve as a map of the family relationships, especially the distribution of power and authority within the family, and might enable practitioners to understand the reasons why particular individuals reject or respond well to agency-formulated vocational rehabilitation plans.

A counselor who reviews the checklist may be able to identify members of primary groups who could work cooperatively with program staff toward the rehabilitation of a client. He or she might also distinguish those persons whose behaviors would inhibit the client's adjustment and recovery, from those whose behaviors would furnish the emotional, physical, and economic supports necessary to the client in order to achieve and maintain rehabilitation gains.

At present, our methods of collecting baseline data on claimants do not give sufficient weight to family structure considerations. The diagnostic checklist would ensure that information on family and role relationships was on record in some form convenient for counselor use. While the costs of introducing the checklist procedure and analyzing the information contained in the lists might be high, they would be offset by the benefits associated with improved program performance. These benefits include greater client satisfaction, more enduring rehabilitation gains, and an increase in the number of successful case closures. Welfare and social service costs would be reduced as more clients returned to work and as the cost burdens that disability imposes upon other members of the family were eased.

A third and related policy recommendation concerns the estimation of costs. At present, closure costs are determined by individual rather than by family (or primary group) performance. Because the economic consequences of disability are felt by all members of the group, however, it would be advisable to evaluate the costs and benefits of rehabilitation in terms of the group rather than the individual at risk. When a worker becomes disabled, he or she and the family may be forced to rely on welfare or some form of income support. Alternatively, another family member may have to go to work to recover the wage income lost through disability. A third possible outcome would be for a nondisabled working member of the family to retire from the labor force and give up his or her income in order to care for a disabled family member in the home. Adjustments and compensations of this kind within the household underscore the wisdom of treating rehabilitation costs in terms of the family or primary group.

Pilot Programs in Utilization of Human Relations and Teaching Skills of Family Members

Because of the close association and interaction of individuals within a family, the family group is well-suited to assist in the care, treatment, and skill training of any member who becomes disabled. Until recently, however, agency professionals have not attempted to make use of the human relations skills and teaching capabilities that many families possess. Instead, as the population in need of rehabilitation services grows and as demand increases, government has responded by developing more extensive public support systems for claimants. This policy has led to increased capital investments in public agencies, expansion of the pool of service professionals and paraprofessionals, and larger operating budgets.

There are a number of ways in which government might avail itself of the resources offered by the family. Family members might be trained as home health aides and skilled chore workers. Programs to enhance and develop the human relations skills of family members could be designed and carried out with the cooperation and assistance of service professionals. The objective of such programs would be to give the individual family member the counseling skills he or she needs to help the rehabilitation client find a job and to help the family as a whole maintain morale and develop interpersonal competence. The contributions of these lay trained persons need not be limited to their own family; if they prove to be effective rehabilitation workers within the household, then they might be employed to work with clients who are not members of families or closely knit groups.

The training of voluntary family workers may have positive or negative effects upon current vocational rehabilitation structures and programs. As an auxiliary cadre of workers, these volunteers can provide services "on call." The introduction of these workers into the rehabilitation process may reduce the actual workload of the rehabilitation professionals, at the same time it asks more of them in a supervisory capacity. Job definitions and philosophies of practice might eventually be affected, and the professionals might experience some erosion of their status and authority.

Service and Financial Supports to Households of Severely Disabled Persons

The impact of acute and chronic illness upon the financial status and life-style of the family has been well documented. In the overwhelming majority of cases, it has largely a negative impact. It is the family that is given the major legal responsibility for its members and is asked to handle the problems of its dependents.

Because the task of coping with the poor health of family members so frequently falls within the nuclear unit,[46] policymakers should consider methods of assisting those families who take on or are given the major responsibility for the long-term care of their severely disabled members. Some economic supports are available to these families now, but others might be authorized, including rental allowance or property tax deductions, food stamps, income tax deductions, low-cost loans, or monthly cash supplements. Chore and homemaking services and medical care might be made available to these families as well.

The provision of such supports to the households of disabled persons may eliminate certain institutional costs. Other potential benefits are high rehabilitation completion rates, reduced job loss and drop-out rates in the postrehabilitation period, and decreased family dependency upon society's institutions. The net financial effect would be a reduction in third-party costs for major income maintenance and other supportive services. A second but equally important effect might be a substantial improvement in the quality of life for the families of disabled persons.

Rewards for Training and Placement of the Severely Disabled

The financial policy recommendation that this chapter will offer concerns the rehabilitation of the severely disabled. The current rehabilitation legislation states very clearly that the most severely disabled are expected to undergo vocational training and to work toward vocational objectives. Section 401 of the 1973 Rehabilitation Act in fact gives priority to the members of this group. Despite the legislative intent, however, fewer of the severely disabled than the nonseverely disabled obtain vocational rehabilitation and entry into the work force.

Admission of the severely disabled into the rehabilitation system will not occur readily or systematically until providers have better incentives to take on the tough and almost impossible cases. Comprehensive services are necessary to prepare the severely disabled for job placement, and while these are authorized in the legislation, they have not been well funded. Even if an agency invests in preparing a severely disabled individual to the point where he can enter a vocational rehabilitation track and emerge with good prospects for gainful employment, it will receive little compensation or credit for its costly undertaking.

Rehabilitation policy clearly must be revised to "put teeth" into the 1973 legislation. Specifically, the current practice of allocating funds in relation to the number of case closures should be discontinued and replaced by a "weighted case closure" system. Under this system, rehabilitation agencies would be reimbursed at the highest rate for the toughest cases. The successful handling of such a case would involve training a severely disabled person for entry into the work force and placing him or her in a competitive job. The more successful an agency is in getting such jobs for the severely injured rehabilitee, the greater the financial reimbursement it would receive. Secondary rewards for agency personnel who place difficult cases might include an advance in status and greater personal job satisfaction.

An alternative method of ensuring that the rehabilitation needs of the severely disabled are met would be the third-party contract. Rehabilitation program personnel might contract with such third-party agencies as employment counselors or job placement specialists to provide the services necessary to rehabilitate their severely disabled clients. Fees could be scaled according to job level placement, wages, and work stability. Providing such rewards over time would be an appropriate incentive for the job experts to continue their interest in the severely disabled worker and to monitor the worker's progress.

Demonstration projects would be necessary to test the effectiveness of both policy options. Demonstrations of the weighted case closure system would also enable policymakers to work out appropriate formulas for reimbursing those agencies that cream off the best cases for rehabilitation and those agencies that take on the more difficult, severely disabled clients.

NOTES

1. Robert A. Scott, *The Making of Blind Men* (New York: Russell Sage Foundation, 1969).
2. S. Wolfe, et al., *The Meharry College Study of Current Needs for Health and Welfare Services, Phase I: The 1972–1973 Study* (Nashville, Tenn.: Meharry Medical College, Center for Health Care Research, 1974), p. 40.
3. U.S., Department of Health, Education, and Welfare, Social Security Administration, Division of Disability Studies, "Rehabilitation of Disabled Adults," unpublished paper by Ralph Treitel (1976), p. 28. Treitel bases his analysis on the responses to those questions in the 1972 Survey of Disabled and Nondisabled Adults that relate to the receipt of rehabilitation services.
4. U.S. DHEW, SSA, Division of Disability Studies, p. 28. Treitel adds a cautious note on the large proportions of severely disabled turned away after seeking rehabilitation services by indicating that sampling variability may account for the percentage distributions. Also, the base is small and the standard error of the estimates is over 5 percent.
5. Majorie Smith Mueller and Robert M. Gibson, "National Health Expenditures, Fiscal Year 1975," *Social Security Bulletin* (U.S., Department of Health, Education, and Welfare), Vol. 39, No. 2 (1976), pp. 3–20.
6. *Social Security Administration Bulletin* (Department of Health, Education, and Welfare), May 13, 1975.

7. Paul Glasser, "The Family and the Crisis of Health Care" (plenary session address to the Groves Conference on Marriage and the Family, Kansas City, 1976) (Mimeo).
8. U.S. Department of Health, Education, and Welfare, Rehabilitation Services Administration, *Statistical History, Federal-State Program of Vocational Rehabilitation, 1920–1969* (Washington, D.C.: U.S. Government Printing Office, 1970); and Rehabilitation Services Administration, *State Vocational Rehabilitation Fact Sheet Booklet* (Washington, D.C.: U.S. Government Printing Office, 1974).
9. Monroe Berkowitz, William G. Johnson, and Edward H. Murphy, *Public Policy Toward Disability* (New York: Praeger, 1976), p. 38.
10. U.S., Department of Health, Education, and Welfare, "Executive Summary," *The Forward Plan for Health for Fiscal Years 1976–1980* (Washington, D.C.: U.S. Government Printing Office, 1975).
11. Marjorie Smith Mueller, "Private Health Insurance in 1973: A Review of Coverage, Enrollment, and Financial Experience," *Social Security Bulletin* (U.S., Department of Health, Education, and Welfare), Vol. 38, No. 2 (1975), pp. 21–40.
12. Glasser (1976).
13. 40 C.F.R. 229 (1975).
14. U.S., DHEW, SSA, Division of Disability Studies.
15. U.S., DHEW, SSA, Division of Disability Studies, Table 1.
16. Saad Z. Nagi, *Disability and Rehabilitation: Legal, Clinical and Self-Concepts and Measurement* (Columbus, Ohio: Ohio State University, 1969). See also Saad Z. Nagi, "Some Conceptual Issues in Disability and Rehabilitation," in Marvin B. Sussman (ed.), *Sociology and Rehabilitation* (Washington, D.C., American Sociological Association, 1965), pp. 100–113.
17. William Gellman, "The Obstacles Within Rehabilitation and How to Overcome Them," *Journal of Rehabilitation*, Vol. 33, No. 1 (1967), pp. 41–44.
18. Bert N. Adams, *The American Family: A Sociological Interpretation* (Chicago: Markham Publishing Co., 1971); Bernard B. Farber, *Family and Kinship in Modern Society* (Glenview, Ill.: Scott, Foresman and Co., 1973); Theodore J. Litman, "The Family as a Basic Unit in Health and Medical Care," *Social Science and Medicine*, Vol. 8, Nos. 9–10 (1974) pp. 495–519; Ethel Shanas, "Family Help Patterns and Social Class in Three Countries," *Journal of Marriage and the Family*, Vol. 29, No. 2

(1967), pp. 257–266; and Marvin B. Sussman, "The Urban Kin Network in the Formulation of Family Theory," in R. Hill and R. Konig (eds.), *Families in East and West: Socialization Process and Kinship Ties* (Paris: Mouton, The Hague, 1970), pp. 481–503.

19. On the importance of the "everyday family," see Ben Bursten, "Family Dynamics and Illness Behavior," *GP*, Vol. 29, No. 5 (1964), pp. 142–145; Sydney H. Croog, Alberta Lipson, and Sol Levine, "Help Patterns in Severe Illness: The Roles of Kin Network, Non-Family Resources, and Institutions," *Journal of Marriage and the Family*, Vol. 34, No. 1 (1972), pp. 32–41; Marvin B. Sussman, "The Disabled and the Rehabilitation System," in G.L. Albrecht (ed.), *Socialization in the Disability Process* (Pittsburgh: University of Pittsburgh, 1976) pp. 223–246; and Clark E. Vincent, "Family Spongia: The Adaptive Function," *Journal of Marriage and the Family*, Vol. 28 (1966), pp. 29–36.

20. Marvin B. Sussman, "What Every School Principal Should Know About Families: An Immodest Proposal," *The National Elementary Principal*, Vol. 55, No. 5 (1976), pp. 32–41.

21. Robert R. Bell, "The Impact of Illness on Family Roles," in Jeannette R. Folta and Edith S. Deck (eds.), *A Sociological Framework for Patient Care* (New York: Wiley, 1966), pp. 177–190; Betty E. Cogswell, "Variant Family Forms and Life Styles: Rejection of the Traditional Nuclear Family," *The Family Coordinator*, Vol. 24, No. 4 (1975), pp. 391–406; James W. Ramey, "Communes, Group Marriage and the Upper Middle-Class," *Journal of Marriage and the Family*, Vol. 34, No. 4 (1972), pp. 647–655; Marvin B. Sussman, "The Four F's of Variant Family Forms and Marriage Styles," *The Family Coordinator*, Vol. 24, No. 4 (1975), pp. 563–576; and U.S., Department of Health, Education, and Welfare, Public Health Service, National Institute of Mental Health, J.E. Bell, "The Family in the Hospital" (Chevy Chase, Md., 1969).

22. William G. Johnson and Julia L. Makarushka, *Syracuse Closed Case Interview Survey* (Syracuse, N.Y.: Syracuse University, 1976); M.W. Stroud and Marvin B. Sussman, "Rehabilitation of the Disabled and the Hospital: A Look at the Past and a Glimpse of the Future" (unpublished manuscript), 1974; Marvin B. Sussman and Gay C. Kitson, "Adjustment to Divorce and Consequences for Intervention" (Paper presented at the Southeastern Multi-Regional Conference, American Association of Marriage and Family Counselors, Atlanta, 1976).

23. The Syracuse Closed Case Interview Survey consists of a stratified cluster probability sample of workers' compensation cases in 1970 in New York, Florida, Wisconsin, Washington, and California. The National Opinion and Research Center was employed to conduct the in-

terviews. The response rates are satisfactory for surveys of this type, particularly considering the difficulty in locating respondents roughly five years after the last contact. The response rates by state were: New York, 66 percent (836); Florida, 57 percent (469); Wisconsin, 77 percent (497); Washington, 66 percent (432); and California, 57 percent (745). For more detailed methodologic data relevant to the Syracuse survey, the reader is referred to Deborah Challet, Martin Frankel, and Julia Loughlin Makarushka, "Survey Design: Workers' Compensation Study" (Mimeo).

24. Paul D. Steinhauer, David N. Mushin, and Quentin Rae-Grant, "Psychological Aspects of Chronic Illness," *Pediatric Clinics of North America*, Vol. 21, No. 4 (1974), pp. 825–842.

25. Johnson and Makarushka; and U.S., Department of Labor, *Analysis of Narrative Comments on Closed Case Interviews*, Workers' Compensation Study Research Report, by Cooper and Company, 1976. The Cooper and Company study of workers' compensation claimants is based on a random sample stratified by type of disability; N-1029 located in four major cities in the states of California, Georgia, Illinois, and New York. Nonresponse was approximately 62 percent; this was primarily due to an inability to locate the claimant. Refusal rates were estimated to average 10 percent in all four states. A detailed analysis of nonrespondent cases compared with those who responded on such characteristics as age, sex, percent hiring a representative, and amount of money received led to Cooper group to conclude, "On balance there do not appear to be serious problems caused by non-response bias in the results, certainly few not corrected for by weighting by type of case" (p. 24). A 62 percent nonresponse rate is high compared to the standard 35 to 40 percent nonresponse rate experienced by private survey research organizations at the time the Cooper survey was undertaken. Even though the Cooper researchers claim that their respondents did not differ from nonrespondents in significant demographic characteristics, the reader should exercise some discretion in considering findings based on these data. Since the Cooper group claims that proper weighting has in part corrected for this problem, selective data are presented and a cautious interpretation is urged. For a fuller description of sample and methodology, see "A Survey of Workers' Compensation Closed Claims," draft final report by Cooper and Company, August 2, 1976, pp. 1–21 (Mimeo).

26. The statistical significance of these differences cannot be assessed due to differential weighting of state samples.

27. Berkowitz, Johnson, and Murphy, p. 90. Data on disabled women and their rate of return to the work force is currently unavailable.

28. Berkowitz, Johnson, and Murphy, p. 90.
29. William Bowen and Thomas Aldrich Finnegan, *The Economics of Labor Force Participation* (Princeton, N.J.: Princeton University Press, 1969).
30. Berkowitz, Johnson, and Murphy, p. 91.
31. Robert E. Thomas, "The Concept and Process of Vocational Rehabilitation: The First Twenty-Five Years," *Rehabilitation Record*, Vol. 11, No. 3 (1970), p. 11.
32. J.P. Zelle, "Caucus on Counseling," *Rehabilitation Counseling Bulletin*, Vol. 14 (1971), p. 221.
33. C. Esco Obermann, "The Rehabilitation Counselor as a Professional Person," *Journal of Rehabilitation*, Vol. 28, No. 1 (1962), pp. 37–38.
34. Paul M. Ellwood, Jr., "Can We Afford Too Many Rehabilitation Professions?" *Journal of Rehabilitation*, Vol. 34, No. 3 (1968), pp. 21–22.
35. T. P. Hipkins, "Rehabilitation Has Outlived Its Usefulness," *Journal of Rehabilitation*, Vol. 36, No. 2 (1970), pp. 12–16.
36. Richard E. Hardy and Keith C. Wright, "Professional Quandary," *Journal of Rehabilitation*, Vol. 38, No. 1 (1972), p. 15.
37. Marie R. Haug and Marvin B. Sussman, "Professional Autonomy and the Revolt of the Client," *Social Problems*, Vol. 17, No. 2 (1969), pp. 153–161.
38. June Kendrick and Jack Sudderth, "But It Doesn't Look Like a School," *Rehabilitation Record*, Vol. 11, No. 2 (1970), pp. 28–31; and Carl Gersuny and Mark Lefton, "Service and Servitude in the Sheltered Workshop," *Social Work*, Vol. 15, No. 3 (1970), pp. 74–81.
39. Betty E. Cogswell, "Self-Socialization: Readjustment of Paraplegics in the Community," *Journal of Rehabilitation*, Vol. 34, No. 3 (1968), pp. 11–13; Robert Allen Keith, "The Need for a New Model in Rehabilitation," *Journal of Chronic Disease*, Vol. 21 (1968), pp. 281–286; and Robert Allen Keith, "The Effect of Social Control on Rehabilitation Treatment" (Presented to the American Sociological Association, New Orleans, 1972).
40. U.S., Department of Health, Education, and Welfare, Social and Rehabilitation Service, "People Power: Report of the National Citizens Conference on Rehabilitation of the Disabled and Disadvantaged," 1969.
41. Marvin B. Sussman, "A Policy Perspective on the United States Rehabilitation System," *Journal of Health and Social Behavior*, Vol. 13, No. 2 (1972), 157–158.

42. In this discussion, *individualized written rehabilitation program* is used interchangeably with the term *contract*. This is done without prejudging that the Rehabilitation Act creates contractual rights and is a "legal" form with attendant rights, obligations, and penalties.
43. P. Abels, "The Social Work Contract: Playing It Straight" (unpublished manuscript, 1967), with reference to Ann W. Shyne, "What Research Tells Us About Short-Term Cases in Family Agencies," *Social Casework*, Vol. 38, No. 5 (1957), pp. 223–231.
44. Abels, p. 6.
45. Marvin B. Sussman, Marie R. Haug, Frank E. Hagan, Gay C. Kitson, and Gwendolyn K. Williams, "Rehabilitation Counseling in Transition: Some Findings," *Journal of Rehabilitation*, Vol. 41, No. 3 (1975), pp. 27–33.
46. Paula A. Franklin, "Impact of Disability in the Family Structure," *Social Security Bulletin*, Vol. 40, No. 5 (1977), pp. 3–18.

Chapter 4

PREDICTING FUTURE DISABILITY AND REHABILITATION POLICIES IN THE UNITED STATES FROM THE NORTH-WESTERN EUROPEAN EXPERIENCE

John H. Noble, Jr.

A West German correspondent of mine recently wrote:

> Our Social Security System is in deep trouble right now. It was based on a high rate of economic growth, low unemployment, and rather strong wage increases, none of which is true for some time. Instead of the basic reforms, patch-work is being done in order to meet shortrun problems arising from low revenues. Likely as not, this will be a matter of considerable political controversy before too long. The high degree of independence of the different subsystems makes it impossible to set any overall priorities, and reform consists of filling the holes in one subsystem by creating new holes in another one. Political infighting enters into it, i.e., the shifting of responsibilities between the Federal Government and the State Governments. Rehabilitation activities are, alas, affected by it since responsibility for large parts of it are shifted from Old Age Insurance (which is centralized)

Adapted from John H. Noble, Jr., "Rehabilitating the Severely Disabled: The Foreign Experience," *Journal of Health Politics, Policy and Law* 4 (Summer 1979): 221–249. Copyright 1979 by the Department of Health Administration, Duke University.

> to Health Insurance (which is decentralized) and to Unemployment Insurance (which is strongly centralized). Rehabilitation centers and spas find themselves in deep trouble. It's quite a mess and ways to solve it do not seem in sight.[1]

Except for the institutional details about where responsibility lies for administering Unemployment Insurance, the West German Social Security System scenario painfully reminds us of our own. Just recently, the Congress applied some bandaids to our own ailing Social Security System in order to forestall imminent bankruptcy. The pundits predict that bandaids will not do the job of a tourniquet; that Congress will have to undertake major revisions by 1985 if disaster is to be averted. Even Congressman Al Ullman, Chairman of the House Ways and Means Committee and chief architect of the compromise Social Security legislation that was passed, admits to the need for further revisions.

This lengthy introduction to the subject of this chapter is not a digression. Discussions I had in early 1977 with scholars, ministry officials, trade unionists, and politicians in the Netherlands, West Germany, Sweden, Norway, Denmark, the United Kingdom, and with officials of the Commission of the European Communities, as well as documentation I collected concerning the rapid growth of disability expenditures and the factors thought to influence it, all point to lessons that I believe policymakers in the United States should heed. We should be able to learn from each other's experience, if only to avoid the same mistakes.

Overview of Policies and Conditions

At the time of my visit in early 1977, the countries of Northwestern Europe had all experienced recent rapid growth in the numbers of persons receiving transfer payments because of disability and in the amounts of expenditure. Concern was universal about the economic consequences of these trends. Compared to the United States, the countries I visited place considerably more emphasis on "collective security" and permit much less of the burden of ill health, accidents, unemployment, or low income to fall on the individual citizen. As Table 4-1 shows, social insurance coverage against the major threats to economic security is more nearly universal than in the United States.

Automatic indexing of benefits had been adopted by these countries far in advance of the United States, thus protecting recipients of fixed incomes against the ravages of inflation. But by the same token, my economist informants agreed that indexing was contributing to the rate of inflation, although not to the extent that sudden increases in the costs of such primary resources as oil and steel do. Attempts to do away with indexing seem doomed to failure. At the very time I was in the Netherlands, the Dutch trade unions successfully struck in protest against the refusal by employers to continue indexing wages (with which social security benefits are linked) to the cost of living. Even in West Germany where the hyperinflation of the Weimar Republic is part of national consciousness, my correspondent wrote recently that the government's proposal to abolish the gross wage escalator for pensions had little chance of passing.[2]

The causes of rapid growth in the disability rolls were thought to lie both in the medical advances that prolong life and in the general economic conditions of advanced industrial society that, through increased automation and rationalization of the processes of production, render obsolete low skilled and physically or mentally impaired workers. One of my contacts at GAK, the administrative organization that processes claims for the short-term sickness, long-term invalidism and unemployment benefits schemes for roughly 70 percent of the Dutch labor force, cited mental illness as a major problem of all of the cash benefits schemes. He was of the opinion that the stress of job market competition, as well as the threat of job loss due to lower productivity, were destructive to mental health. Escape into invalidism provided one solution for workers threatened with the loss of work.

Table 4-1 Social Security Systems Compared, 1975

Country	Old Age, Invalidity and Death	Sickness and Maternity	Work Injury	Unemployment	Family Allowances
Denmark	Multiple universal pension, assistance, and social assistance systems	Dual universal (medical benefits) and direct provision (cash benefits) systems; maternity covered	Dual universal (medical benefits) and direct provision (cash benefits) systems; compulsory insurance with private carrier (disability pension)	Subsidized voluntary insurance system	Universal system
Federal Republic of Germany	Social insurance system; special systems for self-employed persons (compulsory or voluntary), miners, public employees, and farmers; separate systems for wage earners and salaried employees with equal benefits	Social insurance system; maternity covered	Compulsory insurance with semiprivate carrier	Compulsory insurance system	Universal system
Netherlands	Social insurance system; special system for public employees	Social insurance system (separate but interlocking program of cash and medical benefits); maternity covered	Social insurance system	Dual industry and general compulsory insurance systems	Dual universal and employment related system
Norway	Dual universal pension and social insurance systems; special systems for seamen, fishermen,	Social insurance system (cash and medical benefits); maternity covered	Social insurance system	Social insurance system	Universal system

(Table 4-1 continued)

United Kingdom	foresters, railroad workers, and public employees Dual social insurance and social assistance systems; optional coverage for self-employed and nonemployed with annual income less than £675	Dual social insurance (cash benefits) and National Health Service system; maternity covered	Social insurance system	Compulsory insurance system	Universal system
Sweden	Dual universal pension and social insurance systems	Social insurance systems (cash and medical benefits); maternity covered	Compulsory insurance with public carrier	Dual subsidized voluntary insurance system and unemployment assistance	Universal system
United States	Social insurance, except for casual agricultural and domestic workers and for limited self-employment ($400 annual net income); voluntary coverage for nonprofit organizations, state and local governments, and some clergy Special systems for railroad workers, federal employees, and many employees of state and local governments	Social insurance systems; medical benefits for disabled and persons over 65 Cash benefits in 5 States (R.I., Calif., N.J., N.Y., and Hawaii) and in Puerto Rico; maternity covered only in N.J. and $250 lump-sum in R.I.	Compulsory or elective insurance with public or private carrier	Compulsory insurance system	Means-tested federal-state benefits program for indigent families with dependent children (AFDC)

Source: U.S. Department of Health, Education, and Welfare, Social Security Administration, Social Security Programs Throughout the World, 1975 (Washington, D.C.: GPO)

One study by the Norwegian scholar, J.E. Kolberg[3] and several others, concluded that regional poverty and high structural unemployment as a result of changing labor markets, shifting enterprises, the pressure of imports, and the world economic recession were causing widespread ejection from the labor force of the less able and adaptable workers. Disability transfer payment programs were thought to provide more secure and socially acceptable, i.e., less stigmatizing, sources of income than unemployment benefits or means-tested social assistance. Officials in Denmark, for example, recognized the disability pension as more humane than continuing unemployment benefits because it enabled pensioners to escape the onus of Employment Office "control checks," which they would have had to endure as unemployment beneficiaries, and permitted them to retire and live wherever they pleased. These officials were of the opinion that such persons had little or no chance of reemployment under the prevailing economic conditions of Denmark.

There was evidence in some countries of shaken belief in the efficacy of vocational rehabilitation and retraining measures as means of curing the disability problem. In fact, some informants entertained the notion that spending large sums on rehabilitation was a waste, since the economy was not able to produce jobs to match the raised expectations of clients, nor to yield a return on the investment. Nevertheless, social conscience drives the continuing investment; for many, memories of how the Nazis treated the infirm and handicapped makes retrenchment unthinkable. Another West German contact, however, recently indicated that some cutbacks have been authorized: there has been a reduction in the amount of money paid to persons undergoing rehabilitation, and a new ruling mandates that rehabilitation measures cannot be applied more frequently than every two years, except under very special conditions.[4]

Documentation by the American economist, Robert R. Haveman, of the net social costs in the Netherlands of providing sheltered work to an increasing segment of the working age population was creating a stir at the time that I was there.

Haveman estimated that the costs of producing the unmeasured economic benefits of sheltered employment were in the order of 7,500 to 10,000 Dutch guilders ($3,000 to 4,000) per year, and questioned whether these costs were reasonable.[5] One Dutch economist was so frank as to deny the validity of sheltered work as a vehicle for rehabilitation into competitive employment. This view is consistent with Beatrice Reubens' observation during a period of European full employment that "the vast majority on created jobs for the severely handicapped do not succeed in obtaining regular jobs," in spite of the assumption that competitive employment will result for many.[6] The critical voices are few, however, and for the most part, the Dutch continue to defend sheltered work both as a substitute for institutional care of the mentally disabled and as a superior method to the dole for assuring to everybody a minimum standard of living. The position of the Dutch on the issue reflects their belief that work is valuable in itself and, as such, a matter of entitlement.

The political problems of alleviating the pressures that are building on disability and related programs in the Northwestern European countries are accentuated by public awareness of many inequities within the existing social security schemes. Women are seeking more equal protection. Alcoholics, drug abusers, and persons perceived as "socially maladapted" want access to benefits. What is more, they are having their way. Changes in existing policies are occurring at a rapid pace. While I was in Oslo, Norwegian officials and the media were not altogether happy with the decision handed down by the Social Security High Court of Appeals, which held that disability benefits must be paid to alcoholics. The Norwegian scholar, J.E. Kolberg, taking as his point of departure the strikingly different disability rates that he observed among the counties of Norway, also expressed concern over the claims that new groups are making on the benefits traditionally reserved for the disabled:

> Centralizing tendencies in Norwegian society create problems both in the periphery and in the most intensely expanding areas.

> There are grounds for believing that "the second set of diners are serving themselves" from the insurance system.[7]

In the context of the holding of the High Court of Appeals, the "second set of diners" are alcoholics. But in other instances they are drug abusers, the socially maladapted, and women.

Of the countries I visited, I was most impressed by the policies of the West Germans and the Danes because they sought both short- and long-term solutions to diminished employment opportunities for the less able. In West Germany, the quota system and fines for noncompliance serve to finance an impressive array of rehabilitation and retraining centers. General provisions for apprenticeship and retraining upgrade the "human capital" of unemployed workers in anticipation of an improvement in the West German economy. To the extent that employers receive subsidy to retain and provide training for otherwise unemployable workers, the politically sensitive rate of unemployment is held down. The Danes, in contrast, recognize the near term futility of trying to move people into nonexistent jobs in an economy experiencing very high unemployment, and so have passed legislation that lowers retirement to age 55 for persons less able to adapt to changing labor markets.

There are, of course, great costs and certain risks attached to such policies. Some of the jobs for which people are being trained in West Germany may be surplus when the world economy improves. Some of the people in Denmark shunted to early retirement, on the other hand, may be needed later on, or they may fail to adapt to retirement and so increase their use of the social services, including health care, for the help that they need beyond the income transfers that they receive from social security. While making these policy choices, the officials and politicians of West Germany recognized the absolute necessity of economic recovery if the cost burden on society of an increasingly large portion of dependent persons in the population was to be sustained.

Nearly every country I visited was having difficulty in dividing the financial responsibility for disability programs between its levels of government. The tendency for one level of government to try to pass the problem or the cost burden on to the next level appears almost universal. Diagnostic labels and eligibility criteria tend to get stretched in the direction of accessible resources.

The concept of "disability" easily lends itself to such elastic usage because it refers to nothing *sui generis*. Instead, "disability" refers to the disruptive effects of pathology, impairment, and functional limitations—singly or interacting—on the performance of the social roles and tasks expected of "normal" members of society. The areas of life activities usually taken into account are self-care, education, family relations, work and employment, and civic and recreational functioning. Age, sex, educational status, income, and other indicators of social status condition and enter, either explicitly or implicitly, into judgments concerning disability. The relativity of the disability concept thus makes it exceedingly difficult for one level of government to monitor the behavior of the next. The hazard, of course, is that as governments and organizations pursue cost avoidance strategies, individuals will get squeezed into "solutions" that do not fit their real needs.

Intergovernmental financing arrangements can encourage disability behavior. One level of government may label unemployed persons during periods of economic recession "disabled" both to avoid politically embarrassing high unemployment statistics and to shift the burden of unemployment compensation or public assistance onto another level of government, whenever responsibility for these programs is divided or the cost-sharing formula offers high enough subsidy. The Haveman study of the Dutch system of sheltered employment, for example, shows a striking increase in the number of program participants whose disabilities were labeled as "not elsewhere classified." The program was originally designed to serve the handicapped, but generous central government subsidy of sheltered employment may have induced municipalities to enroll unemployed persons who were not disabled in the strict sense of having suffered the loss of physical or mental function. This practice of distorting the concept of disability to provide income through sheltered work to the able-bodied unemployed and, simultaneously, fiscal relief to the municipalities is an example of the classic problem of "displacement" that occurs in public employment programs.[8] But in the case of sheltered work, the effects may be even more damaging; diverting scarce rehabilitation resources and opportunities from their proper use may increase the stock of needlessly dependent persons in society.

Lessons To Be Learned

What lessons can be learned from the Northwestern European experience in the rehabilitation of the severely handicapped? Rehabilitation takes place within a matrix of disability policies and, indeed, falls within the whole as one subset. Thus, variations in the structure of the entire set of disability policies can influence rehabilitation service technologies. Some combinations of policies and political-economic conditions may be mutually reinforcing and prove productive; other combinations may simply cancel each other out; still others may be positively harmful to individuals and society.

Policy variables that affect rehabilitation outcomes can be crudely divided into two groups. First, there are those variables that are likely to have an immediate effect on individual decisions to behave in certain ways; and second, those variables that are likely to exert indirect and subtle influences. If disability pensions are generous relative to possible wages, then the pensions act as a disincentive to paid work, an incentive to increased unpaid work or homemaker services, and perhaps are neutral with respect to activities-of-daily-living functioning. Until more is known about the effects of policy variable structures, statements about their degree of influence are necessarily speculative. Theory and fragmentary evidence, nonetheless, compel us to consider how these variables *may* influence rehabilitation outcomes. Table 4-2 lists 14 variables, to which I refer in examining the "lessons" to be learned from the Northwestern European experience. I advance my findings as hypotheses only, derived from a variety of expert opinion, statistics, and the analyses of some European scholars.

The Swiss actuary, Simon Courant, has documented the relationship between *benefit levels* and disability claims: the higher the ratio of gross benefits available from long-term disability insurance to previous wages, the greater the incidence of claims.[9]

Table 4-2   Variables Influencing the Outcomes of Rehabilitation

1. Wage replacement ratio of benefits
2. Criteria for judging disability
3. Community attitudes toward work
4. Timing and sequencing of rehabilitation services
5. Extent of labor market discrimination against the disabled
6. Force of antidiscrimination policies
7. Extent of demand for labor in the economy
8. Organizational pattern for distributing benefits
9. Method or principle by which disability benefits are disbursed: social insurance versus social assistance
10. Income redistribution ideologies and policies of the society
11. Intergovernmental financing arrangements
12. Amount of labor force ejection in the economy
13. Age composition of the work force and of the general population
14. Displacement effects resulting from employment of the disabled

As indicated by Table 4-3, the ratio of actual to expected claims exceeds 100 percent when the ratio of gross insurance benefits to salary reaches 60 to 70 percent, and jumps to 137 percent when the wage replacement ratio rises above 70 percent. Accordingly, restoration to paid work as the result of rehabilitation services is less likely to occur as disability pension benefits exceed 60 percent of wages. Indeed, one might go one step further and infer that the size of the pension should be taken into account when defining the severity of "vocational" disability for purposes of judging "rehabilitative" feasibility.

The *definition of disability* as "total work incapacity" is more stringent than one that tests incapacity only with respect to usual occupation. Countries employing an occupational definition of disability are likely to experience less success in restoring people to work than those that apply a more stringent test of work incapacity as the condition for paying benefits. The size of the wage replacement ratio, however, probably makes some

Table 4-3 Ratio of Actual to Expected Claims by the Ratio of Gross Benefits to Salary: Group Long-Term Disability Insurance with Six-Month Deferment Period, North America, 1966–1972

Ratio of Gross Benefits to Salary (%)	Ratio of Actual to Expected Claims (%)
Less than 50	56
50	71
50 to 60	88
60 to 70	108
More than 70	137
All	83

Source: *Transactions of the Society of Actuaries, 1974 Reports,* cited in Simon Courant, "The Influence of Sex and Government on Disability Experience," Paper delivered at Meeting of the Norwegian Society of Actuaries, Oslo, March 10, 1977.

difference. The definition of disability establishes the threshold for eligibility, while the wage replacement ratio creates a work incentive or disincentive. Other possible influences here are community attitudes toward work and toward income redistribution. A strong work ethic, coupled with stigmatizing or punitive practices in the administration of income transfer programs, may offset to some extent both a lower disability threshold and the attraction of high benefits relative to wages.

The *timing and sequencing* of rehabilitation services can influence outcomes. For example, in the United States under social security, rehabilitation services are paid for only after eligibility for disability benefits has been established at the end of a five-month waiting period from onset of illness or impairment, and we might surmise that the delay in services would reduce the individual's chances for a successful rehabilitation. Similarly, in those cases where the amount of benefits is dependent on the degree of disability and is subject to contest, as in workers' compensation programs or in law suits for negligent harm, claimants may resist or delay rehabilitation until after settlement, and thereby diminish prospects for full restoration to work. In contrast, Norwegian policy requiring acceptance of rehabilitation services before award of long-term disability benefits appears likely to minimize work disability, provided that suitable jobs for rehabilitants exist in the economy. In point of fact, however, the Norwegian policy that provides more generous benefits to persons undergoing rehabilitation has not worked. Because of poor economic conditions, I have been told, the majority of persons undergoing rehabilitation end up on the long-term disability rolls anyway.

Labor market discrimination against the disabled exists in every country that places premium on maximizing productivity. By definition, work disability involves decrements in the capacity to function on the job. In many instances, residual incapacities of various kinds continue to exist after rehabilitation. Employers who hire the handicapped often incur additional production costs by virtue of workplace modifications necessary to accommodate certain types of disabled persons, higher absenteeism due to sickness, and the like. The developed countries have tried a variety of approaches to overcome labor market discrimination. The efficacy of such antidiscrimination measures can be expected to influence the outcome of rehabilitation efforts directed to restored labor force participation. Quotas, job reservation systems, educational campaigns, special projects with industry to convince employers of the benefits that can be derived from hiring the handicapped, and special legislation prohibiting discrimination have all been tried.

The United States has only recently passed legislation that makes it easier for disabled persons whose rights to jobs and services have been infringed to seek remedy outside of the courts. Before this, the only recourse was to bring suit in the courts — a difficult, time-consuming, and expensive process. Now, under the Vocational Rehabilitation Act of 1973 the federal government is required to use the economic clout of its contract and grant authorities against employers and service agencies that discriminate against the handicapped. The federal agencies will have to enforce the 1973 Act rigorously in order to accomplish the goals of the new legislation. Only time will tell whether this approach is any more effective than the quota systems of England, the Netherlands and the Federal Republic of Germany or the Swedish law requiring employers to petition the responsible government agency for permission to fire a disabled person. Of the countries with quota systems, only the Federal Republic of Germany levies a stiff fine for noncompliance. The predictable result of any quota or affirmative action system is to induce employers and current employees to conspire to apply the "disability" label to as many of the workforce as possible in the effort to preserve the *status quo*. My English informants indicate that their quota system in the United Kingdom does not work better.

Little need be said about the obvious relationship between

the *demand for labor* and job opportunities for the disabled. When economies are expanding and labor markets are tight, the disabled are more employable. The vocational outcomes of rehabilitation services are more readily achieved. But during economic recession, jobs for the handicapped become more difficult to find. Even in the Federal Republic of Germany, where the quota system is enforced by fines for noncompliance, there were early in 1977 approximately 40,000 unemployed disabled persons, 75 percent of whom had been able to hold a job before.[10] The city-state of Hamburg met only 3.8 percent of the required 6 percent hiring quota and paid a total of 18 million Deutschesmarks in fines. In excess of 400 million Deutschesmarks in fines have been collected for the Federal Republic of Germany as a whole.

The question of centralized as opposed to decentralized administration of cash benefits and services programs may influence the outcomes of rehabilitation services. Similarly, specialized service delivery and its alternative, integrated services, may affect outcomes. The impact of *organizational patterns* on rehabilitation services and client outcomes is extremely difficult to document. Manipulation of these variables holds great fascination for policymakers. The Danes, for example, are simultaneously decentralizing and integrating the delivery of social services, vocational rehabilitation, and means-tested public assistance. Many specialized rehabilitation centers are being closed in favor of integrated services delivery to generic case loads of clients by teams of caseworkers and consultant specialists. We can trace this radical shift in organization to the desire to make the municipality the locus of integrated services delivery and, in part, to the belief that the family, rather than the individual, is the proper object and unit of treatment. There is also the possibility that cost-containment is a motive. To the extent that municipalities must levy taxes to pay for the cash benefits and services that they provide, they have greater motivation to exercise restraint and assume more responsibility for outlays than they have when their role is simply to make referrals or to demand more and better services from a county or central government.

Certain countries prefer to provide cash benefits according to the principle of *"social insurance"* (i.e., coverage of certain risks as a matter of legal entitlement and the presumption of need); others, according to the principle of *"social assistance"* (i.e., payment only after determining actual need by means of a test of income and/or assets). Social assistance, by imposing tests of income and assets to determine eligibility, has both the virtue of targeting public expenditures efficiently on those most needy and the vice of branding recipients in the minds of many taxpayers as "free-loaders at the public trough." The stigma attached to public assistance causes some persons with legitimate needs to shun it and contributes thereby to the reputation of public assistance as "target efficient." One would think that where rehabilitation services provide the means of avoiding the stigma of public assistance, they will receive higher value; i.e., higher value in countries that tend to impose a means test before granting cash benefits than in those that adhere to the principle of social insurance. This hypothesis, of course, must be evaluated by reference to *income redistribution ideologies and policies*. Countries that view income redistribution as a positive goal may not regard means-tested public assistance as stigmatizing, whereas countries with negative views may look askance at public assistance recipients and create pressure for them to seek escape through rehabilitation.

If health care and short- and long-term disability benefits are available as an entitlement not subject to a means-test, then many potentially disabling conditions can be caught early and their effects minimized. The prompt offer of services may also protect individuals against the severe financial losses associated with long spells of illness. In the United States, employment-linked health insurance leaves persons who become unemployed or who fall seriously ill vulnerable to severe financial losses before means-tested relief is offered. Added financial strain may aggravate and perhaps prolong illness and even impede full recovery. Integration of medical rehabilitation with general health care and short- and long-term disability benefits could, in theory, favorably influence the range of expected rehabilitation outcomes, especially if linked to the vocational rehabilitation and job placement activities that follow the prescription of an individualized case plan. Again, proper timing and sequencing of rehabilitation services would be expected to promote earlier recovery and return to work.

While all these good things might happen, escalating costs will likely result unless there is strict monitoring and control of the price, quantity, and quality of health services and careful case management of rehabilitation services in conjunction with disability claims processing. The evidence from the Federal Republic of Germany is not encouraging. Pflanz and Geissler argue convincingly that despite generous cash benefits and health services provision, the West German health system is in trouble: "A combination of market factors and social policy has contributed to an enormous increase in health costs which, to the public, does not seem to have been matched by a commensurate gain in the quality of health care."[11]

Intergovernmental financing arrangements between municipalities, counties, and the central government can provide either incentives or disincentives to rehabilitation efforts. If, for example, central government matching or cost-sharing formulas for rehabilitation services are less favorable than those for income transfer programs, local or county governments may find it easier to refer the more severely disabled persons to the sources of cash benefits than to spend for rehabilitation. Again, labor market demand and income redistribution ideologies probably interact with these incentives or disincentives, as the case may be, either to amplify or dampen their effects.

The degree of industrialization and dependence on higher technology of the economy, stability of labor force participation, and the age composition of the workforce and of the general population probably interact to influence the process of *labor force ejection* and, ultimately, the success or failure of rehabilitation efforts. Highly industrialized economies dependent on machines and higher technology have less need for unskilled labor. Increased wages due to the improved productivity of skilled labor tend to bid up the wages of everybody. Employers, in turn, seek relief from higher labor costs by further mechanizing and automating the production process. This results in the loss of jobs that are suitable for the less educated and even for the skilled worker who becomes disabled. Also, as women in the industrialized countries give up the traditional homemaker role to take jobs in the paid workforce, competition for the supply of existing jobs is increased, unless the economies expand fast enough to accommodate all the newcomers. Less able workers—men and women—are ejected from the workforce in favor of younger and more recently trained and mobile workers.

B. R. Anderson explains the phenomenon of labor force ejection as follows:

> The speed of the technical development and of economic growth is now so high that the mobility of the labour force cannot bring about the changes (needed to respond to shifting labour demand).... Disequilibrium is the normal state of the labour market.... The contraction in the diminishing trades and jobs is neither followed by a pull of labour from the expanding (sic) jobs nor from a decrease in labour costs. Consequently there is only one way for the economic contraction to break through: part of the labour force is "pushed" out of their jobs. This can be done through dismissals or through changes in working procedures which cause the "weak" persons to increase their sickness absence, or otherwise.... This means that a rise in the number of "pushed out" persons does not necessarily indicate a growing "weakness" (e.g. physical, mental, educational "disability") in the population. It may equally well be an indicator of a growing rate of technical or economic change in the demand-structure of the labour market. 12

Persons ejected from the labor market in this way may be labeled "disabled" with often exaggerated emphasis on the medical factors that use of the term implies. The function of this usage is really to justify payment of cash benefits for short-term sickness or long-term disability, as well as to justify expenditures for vocational rehabilitation and job retraining.

As previously mentioned, the *age composition* of the workforce and of the general population may interact to ease or aggravate the process of labor force ejection and the associated burden of transfer payments for disability. Withdrawal from the labor force is expected when retirement age is reached, but generally not before, except among persons who have attained substantial means or who suffer the misfortune of serious illness or disability. Just about every data source and study shows that the incidence of disability increases with age. The history of the Social Security Disability Insurance program in the United States since 1960 indicates that whatever the time trend, the number of awards per 1,000 insured climbs with advancing age and leaps when people reach the 45 to 54 age bracket. Except in the Netherlands, large-scale withdrawal from the labor force has occurred among men in the 50 to 64 age group in the United States and the Northwestern European countries, as Table 4-4 makes clear. But as indicated by the same table, increased labor force participation by women in the same age group has more than offset the loss of male workers in every country except Norway and the Federal Republic of Germany. Population growth has also played a role in causing a net increase or decline of labor force participants. The influence of this factor is seen most strikingly in the Federal Republic of Germany, where the military and civilian casualties of World War II led to a substantial drop in the total population in the 50 to 64 age group. This is not to imply that all labor force withdrawal is the result of illness or disability or even unemployment; the availability of income transfer payments must in itself be a contributing factor.

The reduced labor force participation of men in some countries may create, by virtue of the need to provide transfer payments to persons who give up work and to offer rehabilitation services to those whose attachment to the labor force is marginal, a greater cost burden for the economically active

Table 4-4 Changes in Male and Female Populations, Ages 50–64, Their Labor Force Participation (LFP), and Resulting Increase or Decline as Ratio of Expected Value of Populations at End of Time Period, Selected Countries and Years

Countries and Years	Total Pop. Increase/ Decline A	% LFP Earlier Year B	No. Expected Workers (A × B) C	% LFP Later Year D	No. Actual Workers Later Year (A × D) E	Net Increase Decline (E − C)* F	Ratio of Net Increase/ Decline to Expected Value (F/C × 100) G
Denmark (1960–1970)							
Male	37,221	93.6	34,839	86.2	32,085	− 2,754	− 7.90
Female	34,299	32.0	10,976	47.9	16,429	5,453	+49.68
Federal Republic of Germany (1961–1975)							
Male	−832,839	86.0	−716,242	78.5	−653,779	62,463	− 8.72
Female	−350,957	31.2	−109,499	33.7	−118,273	− 8,774	+ 8.01
Netherlands (1960–1971)							
Male	1,445	80.9	1,169	85.1	1,230	61	+ 5.22
Female	114,422	13.5	15,447	17.0	19,452	4,005	+25.93

(Table 4-4 continued)

Norway (1960–1970)						
Male	39,824	93.7	37,315	86.7	34,527	− 2,788	− 7.47
Female	35,427	25.0	8,857	30.8	10,912	2,055	+23.02
United Kingdom† (1961–1971)						
Male	403,086	98.2	395,830	95.3	384,141	−11,689	− 2.95
Female	96,622	41.5	40,098	51.4	49,664	9,566	+23.86
Sweden (1960–1970)						
Male	70,845	90.6	64,186	85.7	60,714	− 3,472	− 5.41
Female	60,095	30.3	18,209	39.3	23,617	5,408	+29.70
United States (1960–1970)						
Male	1,891,426	87.1	1,647,432	84.6	1,600,146	−47,286	− 2.87
Female	2,665,787	39.6	1,055,652	45.7	1,218,265	162,613	+15.4

*The net increase/decline represents the difference at the end of the time period of the observed number of workers and the number that was expected on the basis of the earlier labor force participation rate applied to the later population base.

†For the United Kingdom, 20–64 years because of reporting shifts in the age classes of the series; because the series for the United Kingdom does not permit isolation of the 50–64 age group, comparisons with the other countries are not possible.

Source: International Labor Organization, Yearbook of Labor Statistics, 1966, 1971, 1973, 1976 (Geneva: ILO).

portion of the population than in others. Unless the high-risk age group diminishes in number (as in the Federal Republic of Germany), countries that replace men with women on a one-for-one or even a two-for-one basis seem likely to run into trouble. The problem arises because the social security systems of the seven countries under discussion use the payroll tax to maintain "pay-as-you-go" benefit programs for retired and disabled workers, with the exception of Denmark, which pays out of general revenues.

Men qualifying for benefits generally have longer tenure in the workforce and higher wages than women and consequently are entitled to higher levels of benefits. Therefore, it will take the taxes on the lower wages of more women to pay for the generally higher benefits of each man who retires or leaves the workforce prematurely because of ill health or disability. No relief in this regard can be expected from the taxes of younger workers unless their numbers are growing as a result of rising birthrates or labor force participation sufficiently high to offset the reduced participation of older workers. In the case of the countries under discussion, unfortunately, such a development has not taken place. Birthrates have been on the decline for some time now, and labor force participation among younger men has either remained constant or decreased slightly over the time periods of comparison while increasing sharply among younger women. Only if these younger women remain in the workforce and obtain wages comparable to those paid to men, can some measure of relief be expected.

Last in the list of policy variables and political-economic conditions that may influence the outcomes of rehabilitation services is the tradeoff struck between labor force ejection of the disabled and the possible *displacement* effects of their employment. In an employment market where available jobs are fewer than the number of unemployed, simply providing preferential access to jobs for some may result in their gain to the detriment of others with equal or higher skills. To the extent that the less able obtain jobs through preferential access and turn out less work than those whom they have displaced, the economy will suffer a net loss of productivity. This loss becomes part of the social cost of employing the disabled and must be weighed against the entire array of possible benefits to be derived from their employment, including their increased satisfaction with life and their social acceptance by others in the community. For some disabled persons, it is possible that a greater advantage lies in employing more able workers in their stead. The greater productivity of these workers would yield sufficient taxes to pay more generous income transfers to the disabled. Again income redistribution ideology will play an important role in determining what tradeoff is politically feasible. The issue deserves very careful consideration because it means denying scarce vocational rehabilitation services to some kinds of disabled persons. Such a policy should not be adopted in haste. The conditions under which displacement effects occur are not presently understood and may be quite limited.

Predicting Future Policies in the United States

Do these "lessons" from the Northwestern European countries enable us to make predictions as to how the United States will shape its disability and rehabilitation policies in the course of the next 20 years, a period in which the economically active segment of the population will decline, while persons over 62 years of age increase by 24 percent and those over 75 years grow by 50 percent?[13] I think so, and shall make some predictions in terms specific enough to make me, unlike the Oracle of Delphi, susceptible to history's ultimate judgment of accuracy.

Relentless pressure from many provider and client constituencies will prevent the Administration and the Congress from developing a coherent and mutually reinforcing set of disability and rehabilitation policies, responsive to changing political and economic conditions. In consequence, political infighting and a lack of concern for how the different policy subsystems influence one another will promote continued fragmentation and waste of a dwindling resource base. Governments from the municipal level on up will successfully pursue strategies that shift the cost burden of dependency to the next level. Increasingly, the government will create work in both the public and private sectors to meet the rising expectations of the severely disabled. As pressure on the limited supply jobs grows, antidiscrimination legislation will be found wanting as an instrument of public policy. "Earmarking" of created jobs will bring the United States to a form of the quota system.

Despite serious efforts to limit the scope of what is encompassed within the meaning of "disability," the disability rolls and associated expenditures will continue to grow. The failure of rehabilitation efforts on behalf of persons whose disability benefits exceed 60 percent or more of prior wages will provoke, first, efforts to limit the maximum payable benefit to an amount closer to 60 percent or less than prior wages and, failing that, will probably cause adoption, for purposes of judging "rehabilitative" feasibility, of a definition of "severity" that takes into account both the type of impairment and the size of the wage replacement ratio. Individuals whose disabilities are defined as "severe" because they are unlikely to be placed in a job paying more than the net value of the benefit will be considered poor candidates for vocational rehabilitation. The effect of such a policy, of course, would be to limit opportunities for vocational rehabilitation to persons of higher socioeconomic status. The wage replacement ratios for these persons under Social Security Disability Insurance are well below 60 percent, compared to the ratios sometimes exceeding 100 percent that prevail, by virtue of the minimum "social adequacy" benefit guarantee, among beneficiaries whose former earnings were low.

The wage replacement ratios of disabled municipal, state, and federal employees are a different matter. They appear scandalously high at the present time and are getting bad press. Nevertheless, I predict that civil servants in the United States will continue to receive more generous fringe benefits than the rest of the workforce, just as their Northwestern European counterparts have done.

The United States will eventually permit general taxes to supplement payroll taxes as the source of revenue for the Social Security System. This will bring the U.S. policy closer to the progressivism of the Northwestern European tax structures. I do not expect, however, that shifting the tax base to general revenues will make American attitudes towards welfare any more liberal. Americans will continue to evaluate welfare recipients negatively and will expand the means-test, ostensibly to contain costs and to target resources efficiently to persons having greatest need. Such a policy toward the disabled has the bad effect of adding to the burden of disability the stigma of welfare, and the good effect of increasing the incentive for disabled persons to return to work—sometimes even at wages less than the net value of the transfer payment—in order to escape the stigma of welfare. Those rehabilitation services that provide the means of avoiding the stigma of welfare will be favored more by countries that impose a means-test before granting cash benefits than by those that adhere to the principle of social insurance. Accordingly, Americans will continue to support rehabilitation services for public assistance recipients, regardless of their chances of securing substantial gainful employment, and will eventually have to resort to government created jobs and sheltered work to insure successful job placement. As in the Netherlands, however, this combination of rehabilitation services and sheltered work will yield a net social cost rather than a gain if calculated in measurable economic terms. "Make-work" is simply not as good for anyone as work for which there is a demand in the economy.

Notes

1. Personal communication, dated January 15, 1978.
2. Personal communication, dated February 12, 1978.
3. J.E. Kolberg and A. Viken, "Om trygdeforbrukets samfunnsmessige

bakgrunn," in Levekorsundersøkelsen: Uførepensjon og samfunnstruktur, *Norges Offentlige Utredninger*, 1977:2 (Oslo 1977: Universitetsforlaget).

4. Personal communication, dated February 12, 1978.
5. R.H. Haveman, *A Benefit-Cost and Policy Analysis of the Netherlands Social Employment Program* (Leiden: University of Leiden, 1977).
6. B.G. Reubens, *The Hard-to-Employ: European Programs* (New York: Columbia University Press, 1970), p. 212.
7. J.E. Kolberg and A. Viken, Para. 9.1.
8. See D.O. Sewell, "Discussion: Occupational Training Programs and Manpower Programs for the Disadvantaged," in G.G. Somers and W.D. Wood (eds.), *Cost-Benefit Analysis of Manpower Programs* (Kingston, Ontario: Queen's University Industrial Relations Centre, 1969), pp. 160–169.
9. S. Courant, "The Influence of Sex and Government on Disability Experience." (Paper delivered at the meeting of the Norwegian Society of Actuaries, Oslo, March 10, 1977.)
10. Estimates given during a personal interview with an official of the city-state of Hamburg, Federal Republic of Germany, February 1977.
11. M. Pflanz and U. Geissler, "Rapid Cost Expansion in the Health Care System of the Federal Republic of Germany," *Preventive Medicine* Vol. 6 (1977), p. 290.
12. B.R. Anderson, "Sociomedial Aspects of Disability and Rehabilitation." (Section G Position Paper, Fourth International Conference on Social Science and Medicine, Elsinore, August 12–16, 1974.)
13. U.S. Department of Commerce, Bureau of Census, "Projections of the Population of the U.S.: 1975–2050," Series P-25, No. 601 (October 1975).

Chapter 5

PRIVATE AND PUBLIC REHABILITATION
George T. Welch

Rehabilitation has existed both as a concept and as an ongoing program for many years, both in the federal and private sectors. Federal programs were set up in this country over fifty years ago to service disabled Americans. At various times since then, the federal programs have changed their direction and their emphasis. Initially giving priority to the severely disabled, the federal programs later turned their attention to specific types of disability. In the 1960s, the programs responded to the needs of individuals who were not so much disabled as disadvantaged, culturally or economically or in other ways. Now the federal emphasis seems to have shifted back to the severely handicapped. A trend has occurred in quite a few states to place vocational rehabilitation in the position of providing and monitoring all rehabilitation services in workers' compensation cases and in automobile no-fault cases. This move certainly cannot be in the best interest of the disabled, since monopoly from any source will not produce a system of top performance. That vocational rehabilitation should at once provide services and oversee the performance of its competitors strikes this author as unjust. Yet the policy is presently being urged by some, and at great cost to the state/federal system of vocational rehabilitation.

The relationship of the insurance industry and of business in general to rehabilitation has come about primarily because of the financial stake employers and their insurance carriers have in the disability of workers. Some companies, of course, have been involved in the rehabilitation process because they have perceived a moral obligation to their workers—some would term such a concern paternalism—or because they have felt it was good for the corporate image.

In recent years, however, the support for rehabilitation has become a matter of financial necessity for many. The skyrocketing costs of medical care and disability payments have demanded some method by which the insurance companies and self-insured corporations can hope to control those costs. It rapidly became apparent that the primary means of accomplishing this was by securing the rehabilitation of the disabled individual and his or her return to productive work. Rehabilitation was to be undertaken with the specific objective of seeking maximum recovery in the minimum length of time consistent with the well-being of the disabled person.

The insurance industry sensed the need for (1) more imaginative and creative approaches to the problem, (2) the initiation of the rehabilitation process immediately following the accident or illness, and (3) the development of a rehabilitation concept whose primary objective would be the return of the disabled person as quickly as possible to a productive life and particularly to a job. The private sector rehabilitation effort was begun in order to meet these needs. The insurance companies themselves set up in-house rehabilitation programs, and independent companies were formed to provide rehabilitation services to the insurance companies and self-insured corporations. Today private sector rehabilitation is a strong and growing service, and its success attests to the real nature of the needs that it has filled. Moreover, we can be assured that if the rehabilitation industry had failed to supply necessary services, it would, as a private enterprise, quite simply have gone out of business.

The first private sector rehabilitation programs were those of the insurance companies themselves. Many of the in-house programs are still in existence and have a deep commitment in dollars and people. Many insurance companies have even established rehabilitation departments.

The involvement of the insurance carriers and the self-insured corporations is not confined to those cases arising from workers' compensation, of course. They also handle cases concerning automobile no-fault and liability insurance, general liability, long- and short-term disability, and major medical insurance.

The number of insurance companies with effective rehabilitation departments continues to grow. The Insurance Rehabilitation Study Group (IRSG) is comprised of head-office executives from fifty companies who meet regularly to keep abreast of new developments in rehabilitation. The companies they represent write more than 70 percent of all U.S. life and casualty insurance. One of the remarkable things about IRSG is that it embraces life companies and casualty companies, direct writers and agency companies, and mutuals and stock companies. Indeed, rehabilitation brings together representatives from all insurance structures in a sincere effort to introduce a broad audience to the latest and best techniques in rehabilitation.

Following the development of rehabilitation departments in insurance companies, some insurance companies and self-insured corporations expressed the need for independent providers of rehabilitation services. As a result, International Rehabilitation Associates (IRA) was formed, becoming the first organization of its kind in the field. In the fifteen or so years since the first private sector rehabilitation efforts were undertaken, the free enterprise system has done quite a remarkable job. Today, between the in-house rehabilitation departments and the 450 or so independent providers, there are plenty of services available.

The private sector rehabilitation programs were designed to

achieve measurable results in moving a disabled person toward self-respect and a productive and satisfying life. They became convinced that one of the key factors in reaching that objective was a job; that some meaningful work to do every day was the biggest step to a meaningful life.

It is apparent, of course, that the return to work of a disabled person is beneficial for the insurance carrier or the self-insured corporation. But the most important fact is that the return is a boon to the disabled person as well. It builds self-respect and financial independence, leads to an expanded social life, and frees the individual from the loneliness and pariah-like existence of so many of the house-bound handicapped. To use a sports analogy, it gets them off the bench and into the game. It sets the stage for a life of participation instead of a life of withdrawal.

What is the scope and depth of private sector rehabilitation today? Unfortunately industry-side figures are not available, so I will have to rely on estimates and the statistics I can furnish on the basis of my experience with IRA, the largest of the private rehabilitation organizations. There are 450 organizations now operating in the private sector of rehabilitation. At any one time, we estimate that between 200,000 and 250,000 disabled persons are receiving help from IRA's competitors and through the in-house programs of insurance companies and self-insured corporations. IRA has handled over 50,000 cases since it was founded in 1970. It manages the rehabilitation caseload of some 625 client companies, including insurance companies and self-insured corporations.

Currently, IRA is handling over 15,000 cases. These cases are controlled through 40 offices in the U.S. and Canada. IRA does not provide direct treatment or maintain rehabilitation centers. It is not necessary that we maintain such facilities since adequate rehabilitation centers are available. We do, however, refer many cases to the rehabilitation facilities around our country. Our role is one of evaluating, planning, coordinating, setting target dates and objectives, and following through until the objectives are reached.

How does private sector rehabilitation work? What is the state of the art today? The private sector emphasizes treatment of "the whole person," as opposed to exclusive treatment of the person's particular physical handicap. All of the disabled person's needs—physical, emotional, social, financial, and vocational—must be taken into consideration in order to give him the best possible chance to return to a productive life. In the area of physical needs, the responsibilities of the private sector rehabilitation group include the evaluation of clients' physical capabilities and current treatment and the development of strategies to improve those capabilities. Once these preliminaries are completed, the rehabilitation group recommends an intensive medical care program aimed at achieving maximum physical recovery in the shortest possible time.

The mental attitude and emotional outlook of the disabled person are also critical. As part of the rehabilitation process, we attempt to determine the patient's attitude toward his or her future and acceptance of the disability and to assess his or her attitude toward a return to work. We also consider how the patient is disposed toward family and friends, employer and insurer, and the medical and paramedical personnel involved in the case. Our job extends beyond a simple evaluation of the patient's state of mind, however; we also attempt to foster and encourage positive attitudes.

Our experience has confirmed that another significant factor in the rehabilitation process is the attitude of the patient's family. Consequently, we spend considerable time evaluating the family's attitude toward the patient and his or her disability, and toward their own future role and responsibilities. The family's satisfaction or dissatisfaction with the care being provided comes under consideration as well. Finally, we seek to advise the family how they can play a constructive role in the total recovery process.

Disability has important financial implications for the patient and family, and in this area our activities typically include an inquiry into the financial effects of disability on the patient and family, and if necessary, guidance in the budgeting of a reduced income. We can very often relieve concern about family expenses by making funds available through insurance advances or public sources.

Our final area of concern is vocational placement. We are responsible for preparing the disabled person to return to his or her former job and employer. If we find that the client cannot perform all the tasks associated with his former position, then we investigate the possibility of job modification. Alternatively, we can prepare the client for a new job, either with the old or a new employer. Such preparation entails an evaluation of the client's present skills, the development of new skills, and in some cases, full-scale retraining. Once we are confident that the client has the necessary skills, we work actively to place him or her in a new job. If a job for that individual is not available, then we consider the possibility of self-employment. Very often, we are in a position to assist the client in developing the capital from insurance payments and other sources that will enable the patient to become self-employed.

Ideally, the rehabilitation program begins while the disabled person is still in the hospital. At that time, the person is assigned a rehabilitation specialist who will stay with the case all the way. The specialist begins by interviewing the disabled individual and family. It is our belief that this first contact is extremely significant, because no rehabilitation program is likely to succeed unless those administering it have the confidence of the disabled person and the family. It is here that the intensive, flexible, and highly personalized approach of the private sector can make its greatest contribution. Because rehabilitation is underway almost immediately, motivation is kept high and attitudes positive where delay could contribute heavily to a retrogressive attitude on the part of the patient and the family. Because caseloads are kept low (35 or less at IRA) there is personal involvement at a high level by rehabilitation personnel. And most, if not all, of this involvement takes place in the field, not in the office.

Because we get an early start on each case, we can also

control the social and psychological problems that can easily become chronic if neglected. Expert planning and close attention to detail are the essential elements of rehabilitation as we practice it—from the initial evaluation to the process of placing the disabled person in a job suited to his abilities.

Placement is the final indispensable condition for satisfactory rehabilitation. In some cases, retraining of the individual is necessary. It has been our experience, however, that the need for retraining is minimized if the total program is applied aggressively by a dedicated professional. Retraining is the most expensive of all rehabilitation schemes and poses many more personal difficulties for the disabled who must adapt to a new job as well as cope with their handicap. Fortunately, simpler forms of skill development often suffice, and sometimes all that is required to adapt a worker to his or her former job is a slight restructuring of the job, or a physical change in the work environment such as a special chair or work table or tool.

IRA maintains a close relationship with the unique Human Resources Center on Long Island, New York, where continuing research into the vocational aspects of disability has been carried out for years, and where an outstanding library of works on all phases of rehabilitation is maintained. In conjunction with the Human Resources Center, we offer our professional staff the training that will help them to become more effective in dealing with their cases. We call the training program the IRA Vocational Development Institute.

We are realistic enough to know that not every disabled individual can return to work. Our goal when that situation arises is to rehabilitate the individual to the activities of daily living so that a spouse can be freed to work, so that he can have some sort of social life, and so that he can stay out of an institution. Life in an institution is in our opinion the worst prospect for the disabled and for the insurer.

The approach that the private sector takes toward disability differs in some respects from that adopted by the public sector. Many public efforts are aimed at making the disabled person comfortable with his life *as a disabled person.* The private sector wants to help him give up the life of a disabled person as far as possible and lead the life the rest of us enjoy to the extent that he can. In the private sector, there are also significant financial disincentives to prolonging anyone's disability. We are never tempted to delay the start of rehabilitation, and we are alert to prevent the development of chronic disability that may later resist rehabilitation or successful vocational retraining.

The relationship of the private sector and the state/federal vocational rehabilitation programs is at present a problematic one, and it shows signs of becoming even more difficult. As the private sector grows and becomes more efficient in providing services, obviously a potential for further friction exists between the two systems. The state/federal systems may feel that we are encroaching on areas of responsibility they have regarded as exclusively their own. But the private sector services would certainly not have been born, or survived very long, if there were not a need for them. They pay their way, and to do that they must perform to the satisfaction of their clients, the insurance companies and self-insured corporations. We are accountable and we are competitive to a degree that state/federal vocational rehabilitation systems are not expected to be.

The private sector can offer the disabled individual a number of service advantages that the public sector cannot, and it is these advantages that enable us to survive in the marketplace. First, there is no delay in initiating our services. The state programs will only attempt to rehabilitate the person who has already been declared disabled. The disability must be medically stable, or in remission, before they will take the case. Other criteria for acceptance of a case in the state/federal system develop from time to time in the legislative world under which this program operates. The private sector, on the other hand, goes to work at once, and with all of the services required at each stage. This is an immediate advantage; a prompt response improves the injured person's chances of achieving, ultimately, a high degree of recovery. The performance of the public sector is necessarily limited: Someone has said that, like justice, rehabilitation delayed is rehabilitation denied. A further complication is that often states run out of rehabilitation funds by the time they are half-way through the fiscal year.

The private sector has every incentive to deliver the care and counseling needed without regard to the limiting qualifications of time and condition so often part of the publicly funded program picture. The only requirement in the private sector is that the program should move the patient or the disabled person toward maximum recovery as quickly as modern medical and rehabilitation practice will allow. Under this doctrine we believe the best interests of the patient coincide with the best interests of the company paying the tab.

The private sector not only provides care early on, but it also provides all the care that is needed. The patient's entire life can be changed by a severe disability; his or her relationships with spouse, family, and friends, as well as his or her job are typically affected. Outlook and motivation are bound to be strongly influenced by what happens during the early days and weeks of disability; it is during this period that private sector rehabilitation is already underway and the rehabilitation specialist is making on-the-spot decisions that can help immeasurably with the final result. The question arises, "If the states cannot supply services in the early stages, should they have the right to come in on an insurance case and insist on 'coordinating' or 'monitoring' the case after the case becomes medically stable?"

The public and private systems tend to favor different rehabilitation solutions. We think that there could be a natural tendency for the public system to favor long-range training programs for the disabled because these programs are presently available in state-run facilities. Rather than initiate short-range efforts to locate a job for the disabled individual, the public sector may simply fall back on the training program alternative, confident that the slots are there to be filled.

Convenience may not be the only factor that governs the counselor's choice. Some vocational counselors are not really familiar with the world of business where job placement is a priority and where the disabled person's marketable skills must be fitted to available opportunities. Referral to long-term vocational training may seem to be both a reasonable and an easy solution to the vocational counselor, but it may impose some hardship on the disabled person. It may be a way of avoiding, or at least postponing, the tough task of finding a job for the disabled person, and it can also have disastrous consequences for the trainee, who is often far less suited to spending long hours in a classroom than to adapting his or her existing skills to a new job.

The private sector is expert in dealing with the severely disabled industrial worker because that has been its specialty. Its people are experienced in the techniques of handling such cases. Can vocational counselors in the state/federal programs—no matter how dedicated, talented, or resourceful—be expected to have comparable experience with insurance cases? I fear that the counselors may not feel comfortable with this type of case, having perhaps dealt with relatively few of them during the years, and they may not have the medical management and vocational placement expertise required. Moreover, the vocational rehabilitation counselor is apt to have much too heavy a caseload, maybe 100 or 125 cases, frequently more. This permits little time to serve the seriously disabled client who requires intensive casework in the manner we have described.

Can state/federal programs match the accountability of the private sector? And, in fact, is there any meaningful way to define accountability in the state/federal system with its match of federal to state funds? In the private sector, both the company paying for the rehabilitation program and the disabled individual are in a position of accountability. No closure is made without the acceptance of all parties involved, and in case of disagreement, the final determination is made by the courts. The possibility of litigation insures that the programs and services provided by the private sector are both responsible and ethical; thus, accountability is built into the private system. Competition provides a spur to efficiency in the private sector; if you do not do the job you go out of business. I question whether there is similar accountability in the public programs.

The structural differences between the public and private systems may make coordination of efforts difficult. While the two systems have cooperated successfully in the past, some administrative problems have arisen. First, our needs require the prompt response of cooperating agencies and professionals. Our experience has taught us that this can seldom be accomplished as the federal system is now designed. Second, while state vocational rehabilitation has welcomed cooperation by the private sector, particularly in activities involving return-to-work, they customarily require that their own application and administration of eligibility criteria be met prior to providing whatever limited service has been requested. This requirement blocks prompt action, duplicates all the data-gathering efforts, and in effect asks the private sector and the insurance carrier to give carte blanche to the state in the management of the case.

State agencies also insist on the right to "supervise" any case that involves their use of funds. And the private sector professional is refused the right to case data or reports, even when the client has specifically asked that it be forwarded. Some methods must be devised to overcome these and similar problems that presently exist or the two systems cannot work together efficiently and in harmony.

In my view the most important new area of rehabilitation is placement, and I think the private sector is understandably stronger here. We know business and I believe we have the best possible chance to place the disabled person, if it can be done. We feel that rehabilitation is incomplete if a disabled person who could hold a job is not placed. We are judged largely by how successful we are in doing just that. We are not judged by how well we keep the rehabilitation pipeline filled, or how heavily we use existing services.

The growth of private sector rehabilitation seems to have resulted not in a more effective state/federal system, but instead in attempts to make the state/federal system the supervisory and screening agency for providers of rehabilitation services. As the private sector becomes larger and more efficient in providing services, there will be a greater potential for friction as the two systems come into contact. There is already some indication that some people in the state/federal system feel we are encroaching on their territory.

But the very existence of the private sector system is *prima facie* evidence of the need for it. And since we are effectively providing services not available through state/federal systems — at no expense to the taxpayers — I think we deserve the support and the cooperation of the state/federal system. It has become apparent in the last several years that we are seeing the beginning of a taxpayer's revolt against constantly increasing state and federal taxes. As a result, most government departments are not anxious to take on more responsibilities in areas where the private sector is already doing a good job. Unfortunately, rehabilitation seems to be the only field where government is reaching for more power in spite of the increased pressure on the tax dollar — in spite of what would seem to be the need for every available tax dollar to be used to care for those not already covered by insurance. Why should there be pressure to spend tax dollars in an area now being effectively serviced by the private sector and at no cost to the taxpayer?

Through private sector rehabilitation the insurance industry has found an effective means of controlling costs in disability cases. Without this control, the capacity of the industry to write insurance could be threatened. When the industry's capacity is destroyed through continually mounting losses, the consequences are familiar ones: The *Fairplans*, the assigned risk automobile pools, and medical malpractice.

The question arises "Should there be regulation of private sector rehabilitation?" Probably so; we do not, of course, want unqualified or unethical people in our field. We acknowledge also that private sector rehabilitation organizations are not all equal in their performance, any more than state/federal systems are. But in our case the marketplace is very likely to take care of this problem as well. The private enterprise system has a marvelous capacity for rooting out incompetence.

Perhaps the government needs all the funds and people it can muster to work on the cases of the disabled who are not being cared for with insurance dollars and private sector services. And maybe the day has arrived for competition in some areas between the private sector and government. If so, let us be good competitors. And may the disabled be the beneficiaries of our competition.

Chapter 6

REHABILITATION OF THE SEVERELY HANDICAPPED PL 93-112: A RETROSPECTIVE APPRAISAL BY A STATE VOCATIONAL REHABILITATION DIRECTOR

Donald E. Galvin

Some years ago, Pierre Dupont said, "One can not expect to know what is going to happen. One can only consider himself fortunate if he can discover what has happened." From the perspective of a state agency director, I have tried to discover or at least to appreciate what has happened in vocational rehabilitation since the effective date of Public Law 93-112 on December 23, 1973. We in the Michigan state-federal agency have now had slightly more than four years of experience with this law and somewhat less with the amendments. What have our experiences been? Since there have been many players and many developments in this scenario, I would like to isolate for discussion some of the advances that have been made, as well as some of the ongoing concerns and issues in the rehabilitation field. Specifically, I will address myself to the effect of the 1973 law on delivery of services by the vocational rehabilitation counselor and on state agency administration. I will also consider certain developments in the interagency system of rehabilitation that have taken place since the law was enacted.

I will begin my appraisal of developments by relating our performance to our objectives. The Rehabilitation Services Administration states that the goal of vocational rehabilitation is to provide quality vocational rehabilitation services to eligible handicapped individuals with priority given to the severely handicapped leading to maximum participation in gainful employment. The operative words are clearly "quality services," "severely handicapped," and "gainful employment." We want these quality services to be effective, comprehensive, and individualized; we also want them to be coordinated, economical, and expeditious — all this within a responsible and accountable system that respects the rights of clients, providers, and others. Alfred North Whitehead has said that "Vigorous societies harbor a certain extravagance of objectives," and certainly we in rehabilitation have not been modest in our intentions.

I dwell on this point to emphasize that the Rehabilitation Act of 1973 brought responsibilities and requirements more complex and demanding than the relatively simple pieces of legislation that preceded it. The 1973 Act was not an innocent rediscovery of "our roots"; it was not a simple return to a set of priorities and rehabilitation practices the effectiveness of which had been demonstrated long before. Rather, the new law involved new and dramatic elements. There were significant changes in the client groups served by the program, in the manner in which services were delivered, and in the formulation and understanding of agency and client rights and responsibilities. Sections 503 and 504 of Title V, which require affirmative action in the hiring of the handicapped and prohibits discrimination against this group, represented a great advance over earlier legislation and has had a marked societal impact.

Let this report begin then with a consideration of the impact of the law, with its emphasis on the severely handicapped, upon the direct delivery of service by the rehabilitation counselor. Referral development has been affected as counselors in the state/federal program turned away from those agencies who tended to refer disadvantaged clients and looked instead to those agencies who were more likely to refer the severely disabled. For example, DI and SSI disability determination units would have increased importance relative to correctional facilities as referral sources. We in the Michigan state agency found that general public and mass media efforts to recruit a more severely disabled clientele were not cost-effective. What was more effective was simply to inform the appropriate referral sources of the existence of new priorities and case service resources. Demand for services followed, and we simply had to alter our practices, accepting and serving those we formerly denied.

Unfortunately, I must report that in some cases we can not so easily change our practices or so readily achieve success. We in Michigan, for example, have seen a substantial increase in the percentage of both severe and nonsevere clients who continue to be closed as noneligible. "Risk-taking" rhetoric does not so easily overcome decades of caution — a caution still reinforced in case service manuals, procedural releases, and policy decisions. If we consider the interactive effects of the "wise investment" mentally inherent in the feasibility statement, the paucity of available community resources to serve the severely handicapped, the counselor's feelings of inadequacy in dealing with the severely disabled, and the continued resistance of the labor market to the non-college-educated, severely handicapped person, we may have some appreciation of what has contributed to our fairly modest program accomplishments.

I feel obligated at this time to say a few words on behalf of one participant in our drama who, if not overlooked during the last few years, has been somewhat maligned: namely, the state rehabilitation counselor. We bring rather immodest expectations to the peformance of this individual. We ask that he or she possess the diagnostic skills of the physician, the counseling skills of the analyst, the coordination skills of a Hollywood producer, the community organization skills of a Chicago ward healer, and the negotiation skills of a teamster official. In addition, this individual is to possess knowledge of the labor market, career education, social movements, engineering, and special education. The counselors must be accountable to supervisors and empathetic and sensitive to clients, at the same time they are obliged to stay one step ahead of the new computer program that self-righteously records their every case transaction. They are seen by some supervisors as either incompetent and uncommitted or as sentimental, idealistic do-gooders. Clients and consumer groups may accuse them of being insensitive, unknowledgeable autocrats.

In truth, many counselors feel confused, depressed, and anxious. "Counselor burn-out," a popular conference topic, is a phrase that seems to capture much of their feeling. I find it a rather remarkable testimony to the dedication and decency of the state counselors that most have embraced the new directions with the understanding that we were long overdue in committing ourselves to serve the severely handicapped. Most of them are willingly working to learn new skills, to acquire new knowledge, and to examine their attitudes and their basic approach to clients. In recognition of their efforts, some attempt should be made to extend a greater measure of sensitivity and responsiveness to them. Then in turn, they may be more sensitive and responsive to those they serve.

We move now to a discussion of the impact of the 1973 Act on developments in the interagency network that makes up the rehabilitation system. We have found that in many instances, the private rehabilitation facilities that have traditionally been our major partners do not offer the staff skills or the programs to serve the mentally able but severely physically handicapped person. Because of the limitations of many of these facilities, the Center for Independent Living (CIL) movement has emerged as an absolutely essential new resource partner. The centers can provide peer counseling and assistance in resolving housing, transportation, and attendant problems. Perhaps more importantly, the centers provide rich opportunities for leadership development among the handicapped. Center residents have been active in the public and political spheres, as well as working to determine their own destinies, and they are proving to be important role models for other disabled individuals.

The shift in the rehabilitation field toward the severely disabled has been met with the general approval and cooperation of other groups. Most physical medicine and rehabilitation centers, voluntary health organizations, and state agencies serving the handicapped (for example, Developmental Disability Councils) have been willing to assist the state rehabilitation agencies in the design and implementation of joint programs. Progressive state laws and executive orders to benefit the handicapped, enacted in support of the 1973 law, have also helped us to gain attention and response from other agencies such as Higher Education, Adult Education, the Civil Service personnel system, the State Housing Authorities, and private employers. For too long, these state and local agencies looked upon the handicapped as the exclusive responsibility of the state vocational rehabilitation agency. And in truth, because of our ambition, desire to serve, and mild paranoia, many state vocational rehabilitation agencies fostered such a view of their own role. Now with federal and state laws, media exposure, and court challenges, public and private organizations see that they too have a responsibility toward the handicapped. They are coming to terms with the fact that the handicapped are indeed franchised, entitled citizens.

This type of cooperation should, ideally, be pursued on a much larger and more rigorous scale. But the coordination of programs has always been difficult to effect. In the absence of a binding mandate, agency negotiators must arrive at a resource exchange that will work to the advantage of all groups concerned, an arrangement that very frequently eludes us. Perhaps an even greater stumbling block to cooperation has been the inconsistencies and conflicts which become apparent when one attempts to work "within the rules." It is difficult to reconcile some of the provisions of Public Laws 93-112 and 94-142, Title XX, and the Vocational Education rules and regulations. Congress and our federal counterpart agencies must quickly clarify these real (or apparent) conflicts before we can achieve the kind of coordination we desire between state education, rehabilitation, and social service agencies. The system can not operate if we bureaucrats sit in Lansing, Albany, Sacramento, and Austin in fear that an HEW or GAO auditor may see our "enlightened cooperation" as a dreadful or stupid violation of Congressional intent.

Last, let me comment upon the impact that the decision to serve the more severely handicapped has had upon state agency administration. Administrators have seen that the emphasis upon this group and their needs resulted almost immediately in a 20 percent to 30 percent reduction in successful rehabilitants in almost every state and in the nation as a whole. Michigan, for example, suffered a dramatic reduction in "26" closures as a direct result of turning from the disabled disadvantaged, a high success ratio group, to the severely handicapped. A few statistics from the Michigan program are fairly representative of the nationwide experience. Closures went from 12,000 in 1972 (an all time high) to 8,500 in 1975. Further, the success ratio, which was 82 percent in 1970 (admittedly too high, the figure probably reflects low risk taking), dropped to 72 percent in 1973 upon implementing new management procedures that placed value on intakes and plans as well as rehabilitations. In 1976, the ratio dropped even more markedly to 52 percent. We can attribute the decline to the adoption of the severely handicapped priority. But while I have no doubt that the statistics reflect a greater willingness on the part of the counselor to take risks as a consequence of the new priorities, the figures may also indicate that we lack the experience, ability, and resources necessary to do the job. In our state, we recently uncovered two disturbing trends which reinforce this interpretation. First, the percentage of severe cases in service and rehabilitated has plateaued at 48 percent and 44 percent, respectively. Beginning in 1974, when 32 percent of the caseload was severe, we saw a steady, gradual increase to the 46 to 48 percent level reached around January, 1977. Now, however, we see a year of relative stagnation, suggesting that our commitment to the needs of this group may have weakened.

I cannot completely explain this phenomenon. Some in the Michigan agency advance the defense that we have simply been more demanding and rigorous in defining the "severely disabled" and that other state agencies apply the "severely disabled" classification more freely. There is, in fact, evidence that the interpretation of this term varies greatly from state to state. In a recent survey of state agencies, several states expressed concern over the difficulty of identifying the "severely handicapped," some indicated that they had recently made major changes in their interpretations, and all seemed to voice a desire for an improved definition.

Another administration concern that has gained in significance recently is the cost of services. The rise in costs has at least two causes: first, the general level of inflation coupled with the explosion in health care cost; and second, the need of the severely handicapped person for comprehensive and extended services.

In our state, we have achieved full state funding and acquired all the federal dollars to which we are entitled. Yet our purchasing power is at the 1973 level, and we actually have 40 fewer counselors and 100 fewer staff now than we had in 1974. I should also note that our people have been quite successful in the "similar benefit" arena. By taking advantage of benefits and services offered under such programs as the Basic Educational Opportunity Grant (BEOG), the Comprehensive Employment and Training Act (CETA), Social Services (Title XX), Worker's Compensation, Vocational Education, Adult Education, and other services, we have added over $4 million to our $13 million case service budget, yet we are still hard pressed.

I would like to add a word about quality of services and efforts to evaluate program and service quality. As an administrator, I urge that we continue to refine our federal program standards. We also need to improve our casework consultation system so that we may assist counselors to render better, more effective services. We should also develop evaluation systems that will enable us to assess multiple impacts upon clients and to report to the public in a sensible manner in what ways the provision of rehabilitation services made a difference in the lives of those served. The single dimension of success—the 26 closure—may have the merits of clarity, simplicity, and singularity of purpose but such a measure, in isolation, is insufficient when discussing program accomplishments with legislators, auditors, or consumers. It is likewise an inadequate tool for the assessment of counselor performance and has led, predictably, to abuse and misrepresentation by some counselors.

Regarding state and national legislation, I would like to see the state agencies promoting imaginative legislation that would benefit the handicapped, particularly the severely handicapped, in all spheres of their life. While some states have done an excellent job, too many of us go before our legislators with the hackneyed and singular plea for more money and fail to lobby for the type of legislative changes that would bring about improved services and benefits. We have not utilized the legislative process to extend the civil rights, entitlements, and benefits of those we serve.

With regard to independent living rehabilitation, I would simply note that the Council of State Administrators of Vocational Rehabilitation has gone on record to firmly endorse the provision of independent living services. Several state agencies have used a variety of means to establish and extend CIL's and other service programs akin to independent living rehabilitation. We would hope that in 1978 Congress would "let the shoe drop" in terms of extending the mission and objectives of the state-federal effort. We recognize, however, that opposition to a large-scale expansion of the independent living services program exists. Many argue that we should direct our energies to our present responsibilities—providing quality services to the severely handicapped with gainful employment as the objective—before we take on new obligations.

Let me close with a brief review. While I am aware that the state-federal program provided quality services to the severely handicapped long before December 23, 1973, we would be deceiving ourselves if we felt that the Rehabilitation Act of 1973 and Congressional intent simply returned the program to a familiar arena of predictable success. I doubt that we ever successfully served the numbers or proportion of severely handicapped persons that we are now expected to serve. We need, I think, to raise questions about the program and the integrity of its commitment: Do we, in fact, give genuine priority to the severely handicapped? Do we provide this group with the quality services that lead to vocational success and meaningful rehabilitation?

If we are to answer in the affirmative, we must sharpen our skills, acquire new knowledge, examine our attitudes, develop innovative approaches, redirect resources, bring others along in partnership, discontinue some questionable practices, provide expert casework consultation, and evaluate our performance.

INDEX

Abels, Paul, 175
Abt Associates, 114
activities of daily living (ADL), 154
activities of disabled, xxvi–xxviii
Actuary, Office of the, 14–17, 20
administrative approach, 96, 98
administrative conveniences, 26–27, 31, 50, 143
adult education programs, 233, 235
age factors, 58–59, 129, 197, 207
Aid to the Blind, 90, 134
Aid to Families with Dependent Children (AFDC), 137–138, 144
Aid to the Totally and Permanently Disabled, 90, 134
Alabama, 43
allocation of scarce resources, 121–123
allotment plans
 based on rehabilitations, 34–39
 based on savings to trust fund, 43–48
 based on terminations, 39–43

current financing for BRP, 4, 6–8, 10–11, 26
 fixed percentage method, 4, 6–8, 10–11, 26
 proposed financing for BRP, 50–54
American Medical Association (AMA), 172
Anderson, B. R., 206
Arizona, 34, 124

Basic Educational Opportunity Grant (BEOG), 235
Beneficiary Rehabilitation Program (BRP), xxviii, xix, 1–14, 17–20, 24–27, 31–32, 34, 40–42, 45, 49–50, 52, 54–60, 65–66, 68, 70, 75, 81–84
benefit calculations, 20–21
benefit-cost analyses
 and BRP, 15–25
 and return on investment, 113–123

benefit levels, 76–78, 199–200
Berkowitz, Monroe, xv, 1, 109, 114, 153, 168
black lung program, 143
blind, aid to, 90, 134
Britain, 190, 193, 202

California, 35, 43–44, 105
Canada, 218
Centers for Independent Living (CILs), xxxii, 232
clients
  priorities of, 119–123
  relationship with counselors, 151–152, 169–176
  selection of, and incentives, 54–82, 98–99
  served by BRP, 6, 11–13, 21–23
Collignon, Frederick C., 114
Colorado, 34
Comprehensive Employment and Training Act (CETA), 235
Comprehensive Rehabilitative Services Amendments (1978), xvi, xxi
Comptroller General, 17
Congress, U.S., xv–xvi, xx–xxii, xxxii, 3–4, 6, 8–9, 14–15, 30–31, 42, 82–84, 101, 134, 159, 173–174, 190, 211, 233–234, 236–237
Conley, Ronald, 114
constraints, on human services system, 151–158
Consumer Representational Plans, 155–156
Cooper and Company, 165
cost-benefit analyses, *see* benefit-cost analyses
Council of State Administrators of Vocational Rehabilitation, 236
counselors
  and administrative procedures versus services, 26–27, 31, 50, 143
  and client selection and incentives, 54–82, 96, 98–101
  relationship with clients, 151–152, 169–176
Courant, Simon, 197
"creaming," 98–99
criteria, for selection process, 56–58, 98–99

data bases, in BRP, 18–20
definitions, for disability, 151, 158–161, 197, 200–201
demographic characteristics, 56–64
Denmark, 173, 190, 192, 194, 196, 203, 210
Developmental Disability Councils, 233
diaried cases, 18
disability, definitions of, 151, 158–161, 197, 200–201
Disability Determination Services (DDS), 5, 56–57
Disability Insurance (DI), xv, xix, xxviii–xxix, xxxii, 1–10, 13–14, 17–25, 29–32, 34–35, 38–39, 44, 49, 51–52, 55, 57–58, 63, 65, 69, 71, 73–78, 81–83, 101, 118, 133–139, 143, 145, 207, 212, 231
discrimination, 129, 143
disincentive problems, 55, 69–75, 135–136
displacement effects, 210–211
District of Columbia, 34
diversion of funds, 9
Dodson, Richard, 114
Dupont, Pierre, 229

economic factors, *see* financing
educational factors, 59, 129, 197

efficiency, and financing plans, 26–30, 50, 103–108
Ellwood, Paul, 170
employment, and termination, 6, 61–69
equity, and financing plans, 26–27, 30–31, 50
estimates of needs, 108–109
expenditures, of BRP, 10–11, 13
family
  break-up attributed to welfare, 138
  dynamics and mapping, 176–178
  as unit for rehabilitation, 151, 161–169, 176–179
financing, of rehabilitation, xxiv, 1–2, 82–84
  alternative plans, 26–54
  impact of BRP on DI trust fund, 14–26
  improving program performance, 54–82
  intergovernmental arrangements, 4, 6–8, 10–11, 205
  and macroeconomic considerations, 127–132
  overview of BRP, 3–13
  fixed percentage method of funding, 6, 10–11, 26
Florida, 83, 99, 121, 165–166
Ford, Gerald, 155
form SSA-853, 19–20

Galvin, Donald E., 229
Geissler, U., 205
Gellman, William, 159
General Accounting Office (GAO), 17–18, 20–22, 24, 26, 32, 56, 73, 105, 118, 234
Georgia, 165–166
Germany, Federal Republic of, 189–192, 194, 196, 202–203, 205, 207, 210

"handicaps," 158
Harbridge House, 109
Hardy, Richard, 170
Haveman, Robert R., 194, 197
Hawaii, 34, 124
Health, Education and Welfare, U.S. Department of (HEW), 4, 26, 120–121, 156, 172, 234
health care, *see* medical and health care
health insurance, 155
higher education programs, 233, 235
Hipkins, T. P., 170
homemakers, statistics concerning, 109–110
Horning, Martin, 1
households, as rehabilitation units, 151, 161–169, 176–179
Human Resources Center (Long Island), 221

Illinois, 83, 165
impairment levels, 59–60, 158
incentives, and client selection, 54–82
income redistribution, 204
income support programs, 133–135
Indiana, 34
individualized written rehabilitation plans (IWRPs), xix–xx
inflation, affects of, 11, 15–16, 20
insurance industry, and private rehabilitation, 215–227
Insurance Rehabilitation Study Group (IRSG), 217
International Rehabilitation Associates (IRA), 217–218, 220–221

job restructuring, 129
Johnson, William, 153, 164–166, 168

Kentucky, 34, 124
Kolberg, J.E., 194–195

Labor, U.S. Department of, xxii, 115
labor markets, xxiv–xxv, 102, 127–132, 201–203
Levitan, Sar, 89

McConnell, Stephen, 1
Maine, 34, 124
Makarushka, Julia, 164–166
marital status factors, 60, 164, 167–168
Massachusetts, 124
Medicaid, 135, 153
medical and health care, 152–155, 172–173, 204–205
medical insurance, 155
Medicare, 71–72, 83–84, 135, 153
Michigan, 34, 43, 105, 229, 231, 234–235
Minnesota, 34, 105
Mississippi, 124
Missouri, 83
Murphy, Edward, 153, 168

Nagi, Saad, 109, 158
National Council on the Handicapped, xxi
National Institute of Handicapped Research (NIHR), xxi
needs
  estimates of, 108–109
  reduction of, 109–113
  universe of, 108
Netherlands, 190–192, 194–195, 197, 202, 207
New Jersey, 124
New York, 35, 43–44, 83, 165–166, 221
Nixon, Richard, 174
Noble, John H., Jr., 189
North Dakota, 34
Norway, 173, 190, 192, 194–196, 201

Office of the Actuary, 14–17, 20
Ohio, 34–35, 43–44, 175
Old Age Assistance, 134
Oregon, 124
organizational patterns, 203–204

paybacks, tax, 25
Pennsylvania, 35, 44, 105
performance, 54–82, 103–108
Pflanz, M., 205
"pipe-line" problem, 14
placement, as test of program effectiveness, 107
policies, for rehabilitation, 151–182
practitioners, see counselors
Primary Insurance Account (PIA), 15–16, 20, 77
private rehabilitation, 215–227
professionals, see counselors
program administrative reviews (PARs), 33, 56
Puerto Rico, 34, 43, 83

racial factors, 60, 129, 143
recidivism, 21–23
regression models, 65–69
rehabilitation
  allotment plans based on, 34–39
  in Europe, 189–213
  financing of, 1–84
  policy analysis and change, 151–182
  private, 215–227
  versus relief, 132–140
  sheltered workshops, 90, 125–126, 143
  and termination, 6, 11–13, 21–23
Rehabilitation Act (1973), see Vocational Rehabilitation Act (1973)
Rehabilitation Services Administration (RSA), 5, 8, 19, 24, 31–32, 57, 82–84, 102, 111, 114, 160, 230

INDEX 243

relief, and rehabilitation, 132–140
replacement rates, 78–81
resources, allocation of, 121–123
Reubens, Beatrice, 195
Ridge, 109
Rubin, Jeffrey, xv, 1

Schoon, 109
selection process criteria, 56–58, 98–99
service mixes, 123–127
"severity" of disability, 158
sex factors, 60, 129, 197, 207, 210
sheltered workshops, 90, 125–126, 143
Shyne, Anne, 175
slack labor markets, 102, 127–132, 201
social assistance, 204
social insurance, and workfare, 132–140, 204, 235
Social Security Administration (SSA), 1, 5, 8, 14–19, 39, 57, 82, 156, 213
Social Security Amendments (1965), 4, 6
Social Security Amendments (1977), 1
Social Security Disability Amendments (1980), 82
Social Security Disability Insurance (SSDI), *see* Disability Insurance (DI)
South Carolina, 124
SSA-853 form, 19–20
state allotments
  alternative plans, 26–54
  and BRP, 4, 6–8, 10–11
  current plan, 4, 6–8, 10–11
  joint program with federal government, 95–108
substantial gainful activity (SGA), 39, 50–52, 54, 61, 63, 67, 69–74, 76, 82–84

Supplemental Security Income (SSI), xv, 101, 134, 136, 139, 143, 231
Survey of Disabled and Nondisabled Adults (1972), 152, 156–157
Survey of Recently Disabled Adults (1971), 111–112
Sussman, Marvin B., 151
Sweden, 173, 190, 193, 202
system constraints, 151–158

Taggart, Robert, 89
tax paybacks, 25
taxation basis, of rehabilitation programs, 1, 3, 8, 10, 14–15
technology, of rehabilitation, xxiii–xxiv
Tennessee, 34, 124
terminations
  allotment plans based on, 39–43
  from DI rolls, 6, 11–13, 21–23
Texas, 34–35, 83
"time lag" problem, 14
timing and sequencing of services, 201
training programs, 90, 125–126, 143
transfers, 135–136, 143
Treitel, Ralph, 19
trial work periods, 3–4, 75–76
trust fund, *see* Disability Insurance (DI)

Ullman, Al, 190
underemployment statistics, 111
unemployment statistics, 110–111
"unit" for rehabilitation, 151, 161–169, 176–179
United Kingdom, 190, 193, 202
universe of needs, 108

Vermont, 124
Veterans Administration (VA), 93, 100
Vocational Development Institute, 221
vocational education programs, 235

Vocational Rehabilitation Act (1973), xvi, xx–xxii, xxv–xxvi, xxxi–xxxii, 8, 13, 30, 81, 102, 120, 173–176, 181, 202, 230, 232–233, 237

wage-benefit ratios, 61–69, 198
War on Poverty (1960s), xvi
Washington, 83, 165–166
Welch, George T., 215
welfare, and workfare, 132–140
West Virginia, 99

Whitehead, Alfred North, 230
Wisconsin, 43, 105, 165–166
Work Incentive Program (WIN), 138–139
workers' compensation, 143, 235
workfare, and welfare, 132–140
workshops, sheltered, 90, 125–126, 143
Worrall, John D., 1, 109
Wright, Keith, 170

Zelle, J. P., 169